THE MEDIEVAL WOMB

BORDERLINES

Further Information and Publications

www.arc-humanities.org/series/book-series/

THE MEDIEVAL WOMB

HILDEGARD OF BINGEN'S VIEWS ON THE FEMALE REPRODUCTIVE BODY

by

MINJI LEE

ARC HUMANITIES PRESS

British Library Cataloguing in Publication Data
A catalogue record for this book is available from the British Library.

ISBN (Hardback): 9781802700398
ISBN (Paperback): 9781802703771
e-ISBN (PDF): 9781802702224
e-ISBN (EPUB): 9781802703764

www.arc-humanities.org

Printed and bound in the UK (by CPIGroup [UK] Ltd), USA (by Bookmasters), and elsewhere using print-on-demand technology.

Publisher (manufacturer) details: Arc Humanities Press, 14 Clifton Moor Business Village, James Nicolson Link, York YO30 4XG, United Kingdom.

EU Authorized Representative details (for GPSR purposes): Amsterdam University Press, Nieuwe Prinsengracht 89, 1018 VR Amsterdam, The Netherlands. www.aup.nl

CONTENTS

LIST OF ILLUSTRATIONS

PREFACE

WHILE I WAS in graduate school, I suffered greatly with my menstruation. From my undergraduate years, I had wanted to study this subject. Occasionally, people asked why I was studying menstruation, especially in South Korea, where discussing it openly was uncommon. Jokingly, I answered that it was due to my PMS—though in retrospect, I should have consulted an ob-gyn rather than making light of my condition.

My first scholarly encounter with menstruation came in 2007 during an anthropology of religion class, where we read Marla N. Power's "Menstruation and Reproduction: An Oglala Case."[1] Power critiqued earlier anthropological approaches in which many (male) authors interpreted menstruation negatively across cultures. Through her analysis of the Buffalo ceremony—a puberty ritual for girls experiencing their first menstruation in the Oglala tribe of North America—she demonstrated that these rites did not necessarily convey negative interpretations of women's menstruation. Power implied that menstruation cannot be reduced to a single concept of pollution.

This article illuminated for me not only that menstruation and women's bodily functions could hold multiple meanings, but also that there existed a strong interdisciplinary need to understand women's bodies in religious studies. What struck me was not simply that a scholar discussed menstruation—a topic normally deemed "private" and "sexual"—but that women's menstruation could be embedded with various cultural meanings beyond taboos. Power's study profoundly influenced my desire to explore how women's bodies have been interpreted throughout religious history.

My own physical suffering was considerable: heavy flows, extreme premenstrual syndrome. With one week of PMS followed by a week of menstruation, I spent half my life in discomfort. I blamed my female body with its womb, especially as my male colleagues seemed unburdened by such afflictions. I failed to recognize that my body was sending an important message that my lifestyle—insufficient sleep, no weekends, long hours in the graduate office, constant stress—was unsustainable. In Hildegardian terms, my body was manifesting symptoms of imbalance. By the time I took a leave from my graduate program, I was menstruating twice monthly, each time with such profuse bleeding that no sanitary product sufficed even for an hour.

1 Power, "Menstruation and Reproduction," 54–65.

During my semester away, I consulted a physician who was my mother's friend and a devout Catholic. She had visited European pilgrimage sites and offered not only medical treatment but also counselling and spiritual guidance. Naturally, I seized the opportunity to discuss my dissertation topic. Though she might not have agreed with all my perspectives, she listened attentively. One day, she mentioned having heard from God and seeing a fountain in her dream. This reference to a "fountain" startled me, as I had just begun discovering this imagery in Hildegard's *Cause et cure* and *Scivias*. While it would have been gratifying to have my understanding of Hildegard confirmed by the doctor's vision, establishing my interpretation with scholarly certainty required years of additional research.

What remained absolutely clear throughout my graduate studies was the consistent presence of women who supported me through various health issues. My friend C supplied cranberry juice when I suffered from cystitis during a visit to Taiwan. My childhood friend M sent dried mugwort tablets from South Korea when my menstruation would not cease. Y shipped various health supplements, lamenting the inadequacies of American healthcare. These women's assistance helped me envision Hildegard's era, when women necessarily supported one another in the absence of modern medicine. This book represents my attempt to express gratitude to these women.

I am deeply indebted to my advisors and professors at Rice University as well as Seoul National University. Where else could I have discovered such a perfect topic within religious studies? Particular thanks go to my exceptional Ph.D. advisor, Claire Fanger. I am grateful for everything you offered, including our shared experience of sampling mugwort tea. I learned immensely from you and cherish our times writing, eating, and enjoying coffee and tea together.

I appreciate my parents. As the daughter of a church minister and a nurse, with a pharmacist sister, it seems almost inevitable that I would become a joint professor in the Department of Religion and Medical Humanities at Montclair State University. The Religion Department and the College of Humanities and Social Science at Montclair generously supported work on this book, including its Open Access publication. I am grateful to my dear colleagues at Seoul National University, Rice University, and now Montclair State University. Thanks also to P for persistently encouraging me to transform my thesis into a book. Finally, I thank every woman who helps and cares for herself and others. This book exists because of your labour, whatever form of care you have provided to the world.

INTRODUCTION

WEAKNESS. VULNERABILITY. SOFTNESS. Susceptibility. Receptibility. Versatility. Fickleness. Talkativeness. Passivity. Airiness. Permeability. Emptiness. Throughout history, women's bodies have been described as weak, soft, leaky, and open to outside influences. These ideas of "porosity"—their bodies' openness to flows and external forces—appear repeatedly in medieval European medical texts, religious writing, and literature. Often, these descriptions supported negative views of women as physically and morally inferior, which has contributed to modern understandings and treatment of women. Yet what if these same qualities could be seen not as weakness but as sources of salvation, healing, and divine connection?

This book examines how Hildegard of Bingen (1098–1179), a remarkable twelfth-century German Benedictine nun, healer, and visionary, transformed traditional ideas about women's bodies. Rather than accepting the conventional view that women's physical nature made them lesser beings, Hildegard reinterpreted and reimagined female porosity as a sacred gift and healing power, a divine channel through which healing and salvation could flow. In Hildegard's writings, women's bodies appear as fountains, vessels, gardens, and wombs, images rich with both natural and spiritual meanings. These were not merely poetic or analogical comparisons; they reflect Hildegard's understanding of the female body as a site where divine and physiological communication occurs. In her medical work *Cause et cure* and her visionary text *Scivias*, Hildegard presents the female body, especially the womb, as a vessel ordained by God to receive, transform, and create life. Through this perspective, she reframed traditional associations of women with weakness and danger, offering instead a vision of purification, healing, salvation, and spiritual authority.

There are some major differences from the tradition in the way Hildegard of Bingen treats the woman's reproductive body. Drawing on her gynaecological and theological writings, I show how she offers a distinctive example of a female writer representing women's bodies as having beneficial and positive powers. I thus focus on the womb and women's reproductive bodies as the core of understanding women in medieval culture from both men's and women's perspectives, contrasting Hildegard's theories of women's reproductive bodies with male-centred views handed down by the traditions of medicine and theology she learned. I argue that Hildegard represents the "womanly" body (despite its weakness) as having beneficial aspects not given to males because of the purgative and re-creative power of the womb. While she is neither the first nor the only theorist who sees the womb and women's reproductive role as the core of gender difference, I present her as one among few scholars who emphasize women's reproductive organs as having important, divinely ordained functions. I contrast her to many medieval theologians, who insist that feminine reproductive processes are a punishment brought on by Eve's fall, and many medieval physicians, who see them as evidence of women's inferior bodies. I support my argument by drawing mainly on two of Hildegard's writings, *Scivias* and *Cause et cure*.

Here, my aim is not to represent her as a proto-feminist or her views as liberating women. Hildegard of Bingen still heavily depends on the contemporary stereotypical gender roles of her time, such as the popular image of females as the weaker and inferior sex, when she explains the creation and bodily conditions of human beings. However, it is noteworthy that she was not a woman who exactly fit the medieval gender stereotypes. Above all, Hildegard of Bingen was not a weak woman. Despite ecclesial limitations and difficulties imposed on her due to her femaleness, she was someone given to raising her voice in theological and political matters, as seen in her extensive correspondence with clerical and political authorities who sought her opinions. Her influence was more significant than was common among medieval women, though there are a few other cases found among saintly women who spoke from the authority of visions and mystical experience.

Hildegard of Bingen was neither a wife nor a mother, which were the roles expected of medieval women. She was brought up in religious life from an early age and remained celibate throughout her life. Nevertheless, she showed sympathy to women who were wives and mothers, understanding their reproductive processes and functions. As an older nun, she provided care for women in childbirth and remedies for menstrual pains and problems. We find no instances where Hildegard treated menstruation, conception, or childbirth as polluting or as dangerous to males, though it was common to find these attitudes in men's writing. These less judgmental views were based on Hildegard's fundamentally optimistic position that all men and women were created with a divine purpose by God to engage in roles that were not just hierarchical but, importantly, complementary to each other.

I build upon the work of certain pioneers in medieval women's historical studies to support this positive depiction of the woman's body and religious role. Caroline Walker Bynum opens the gate for the study of medieval women by showing how women's religiosity and devotional practices need to be investigated separately, alongside those of medieval men.[1] Barbara Newman continues to be the most important writer about Hildegard of Bingen's theology of the feminine.[2] Monica Green has shown in many studies that medieval medical culture was not entirely controlled by men but also included important contributions by women.[3] Ruth Mazo Karras investigates how medieval women are understood, showing how, despite prevalent misogyny, they contribute to, as well as participate in, society and culture.[4] And Dyan Elliot emphasizes how women's weakness and porosity transformed into the possibility of receiving the Holy Spirit.[5]

This book differs from the work of these major historians by its narrow focus on one material and conceptual aspect of the distinction between women and men: the womb and its functions, representing woman's porosity. By the conclusion of this book, I hope to show how Hildegard of Bingen appreciates women's reproductive bodies and their functions as important small mirrors of God's creation and salvation. Granted that the Virgin Mary's womb was already understood as an important object of praise for its role in bringing Jesus into this world, I suggest that Hildegard of Bingen also writes about ordinary women while emphasizing the positive meanings and divine powers attributed to the womb and the female reproductive body. Even when Hildegard follows the traditional notion of women as the weaker sex, she manages to create positive interpretations. Ultimately, she always manages to show that God made women in this way for good reason, thus converting the things that were traditionally treated as signs of women's inferiority into strong points in her well-integrated discussions of female physiology and theology.

The degree to which women's reproductive bodily processes, such as menstruation and childbirth, were viewed with negative connotations, as signs of inferiority, impurities, or toxins, is hard to overestimate. In the Vul-

---

1 Bynum, *Holy Feast and Holy Fast*; Bynum, *Wonderful Blood*.

2 Newman, *Sister of Wisdom*; Newman, "Hildegard and Her Hagiographers," 16–34.

3 Green, *Making Women's Medicine Masculine*; Green, "In Search of an 'Authentic' Women's Medicine," 25–54.

4 Karras, *Sexuality in Medieval Europe*.

5 Elliot, "Gender and the Christian Traditions," 21–35.

gate, attitudes to menstruation can be seen in the prophecy of Isaiah for people living against God's will, "And thou shalt defile the plates of thy graven things of silver, and the garment of thy molten things of gold, and shalt cast them away as the uncleanness of a menstruous woman. Thou shalt say to it: Get thee hence" (Isaiah 30:22).[6] This use of the menstrual-cloth metaphor shows how deeply ingrained such negative attitudes were.

However, these traditional attitudes do not mean that only unfavourable attitudes towards women's bodies and reproductive symptoms existed in the Middle Ages. Although male authors tended to dominate intellectual, medical, and religious spheres, which is not surprising in a male-centred society, I focus on Hildegard of Bingen as a woman professionalized in gynaecological and theological knowledge who promoted positive understandings of the womb and reproduction by highlighting the porous nature of women. I would like to show that Hildegard not only receives conventional representations of the woman's body but also, as a woman, uses them, even manipulates them, in woman-friendly ways by emphasizing women's purgative and re-creative bodies in both her medical and her theological accounts.

After showing Hildegard's medieval understanding of the woman's porous body, I end this book with a case study of Korean women's folk medicine, which also highlights the porosity of the female body. In presenting the porous female body not as a flaw but as a site of divine interaction, Hildegard offers a powerful reimagining of gender, medicine, and theology. This book seeks to recover and amplify that vision for both historical understanding and contemporary thought. Therefore, this book also draws a line from Hildegard's reflections to modern Western and non-Western alternative and folk medicine to show how the porosity of female bodies remains important.

---

6 English translation from the Douay-Rheims Bible. The Latin is "et contaminabis lamminas sculptilium argenti tui et vestimentum conflatilis auri tui et disperges ea sicut inmunditiam menstruatae egredere dices ei." Also, Isaiah 64:6 presents a similar analogy between menstruating women and sinners in the context of repentance: "And we are all become as one unclean, and all our justices as the rag of a menstruous woman: and we have all fallen as a leaf, and our iniquities, like the wind, have taken us away." The Latin is "et facti sumus ut inmundus omnes nos quasi pannus menstruatae universae iustitiae nostrae et cecidimus quasi folium universi et iniquitates nostrae quasi ventus abstulerunt nos."

Woman's Porous Body as Devil's Gateway

In this book, I conceptualize a vessel's capacity for flow as permeability or porosity, drawing from Hildegard's medical and religious terminology. The womb is frequently characterized as a vessel in medieval texts, just as women themselves are often described as vessels. While Hildegard recognizes this porosity as a potential power for maintaining or restoring health, historically and traditionally, the same quality has frequently been deployed against women as evidence of their inferiority. To appreciate the revolutionary nature of Hildegard's positive reinterpretation of the female porous body, it is essential to first examine how pervasively and dauntingly negative the traditional characterizations were.

In the history of medicine, women have consistently been relegated to a passive position, characterized primarily by their capacity to "receive something." Aristotle emphasized that men are active in the reproductive process, while women are passive.[7] Even Galen, despite advancing the more balanced two-seed theory, maintained that women played a comparatively passive role in conception, with their contribution considered weaker and less vital than the male seed.[8] This passivity is also found in the works of Thomas Aquinas: "[a]mong perfect animals the active power of generation belongs to the male sex, and the passive power to the female."[9] This passivity is related to the weakness that women were assumed to have. Earlier than Aquinas, Isidore of Seville claims that the man's power (Latin *uis*) is shown in the Latin word *uir*, while the woman or *mulier* has the softness expressed by *mollier*.[10] For him, those etymologies justified the claim that women are meant to be subjected to men, who are stronger and unbreakable.

At the same time, this porosity is understood as being easily defeated by evil or spiritually contaminated. Women were believed to corrupt others

---

7 Aristotle, *De generatione animalium*, trans. Platt, bk. 1, chap. 20, §§27–32, p. 729a.

8 Galen, *On the Usefulness of the Parts of the Body*, trans. Tallmadge, bk. 14, chap. 2.296, §5, p. 628.

9 Thomas Aquinas, *Summa theologiae*, trans. Fathers of the English Dominican Province, pt. 1, q. 92, "The Production of the Woman," article 1, https://www.newadvent.org/summa/1092.htm. See also article 2, "Defuisset enim bonum ordinis in humana multitudine si quidam per alios sapientiores gubemati non fuissent. Et sic ex tali subjectione naturaliter femina subjecta est viro, quia naturaliter in homine magis abundat discretio rationis."

10 Isidore of Seville, *Etymologiarum sive originum libri XX*, ed. Lindsay, bk. 11, pt. 2, 1:17–20.

easily as much as they can be easily corrupted.[11] In the moral view of medieval Christianity, Eve is the exemplar of how women's fleshy and porous bodies brought sin into the world. Eve's weakness causes her to succumb to the serpent's temptation, bringing death to human beings. As punishment, Eve's body and those of her female descendants became even weaker, receiving the flow of menstruation and reproductive processes.

These perceptions of a woman's body are closely interwoven with both medical and religious understandings. When certain medical ideas, widely accepted as "scientific," are used to explain a woman's overflowing sexuality, it becomes evident that religious language not only has the potential to take advantage of women but, in a sense, is required to do so. When gaps are found in medical knowledge about a woman's biological body, religious meanings could fill those gaps, and vice versa. When a specific idea is widely accepted as true, both religion and medicine are often expected to explain it.

A woman's sexuality also plays an important role in understanding her fleshy nature. In order to verify their medical ideas in religious terms, theologians sought reasons from Genesis, in the idea, for example, that Eve is born out of the body of Adam, which makes her more physical and therefore causes her body to contain a stronger physical desire.[12] At the same time, the description of Eve succumbing to the deceptive plan of the serpent in scripture could be used as religious proof that women are more lustful than men. Similarly, physicians could use this reasoning to explain that the sexual drives of women are more powerful, using different means but coming to the same conclusion.

This concept of female porosity was also applied to "effeminate" men who, despite being physiologically male, were not considered sufficiently masculine to receive equal treatment as men. In medieval Christian polemic, Jews and Muslims were characterized as "less complete" through accusations of effeminacy. This gendered discourse served to position non-Christian males as fundamentally inferior. Notably, this rhetoric extended to attributing female biological processes to Jewish men, who were claimed

11 In her analysis of Heloise's letters to Abelard, Karma Lochrie identifies Heloise's evident concern regarding female homoeroticism between religious and secular women with "foulness of a corrupted mind," a subject systematically overlooked by her male theological contemporaries and subsequently neglected in modern scholarly discourse. Lochrie, *Heterosyncrasies*, 33.

12 Karras, *Sexuality in Medieval Europe*, 4.

to suffer from bloody flux or menstruation[13]—a physiological impossibility that nonetheless reinforced their perceived deviation from Christian masculine ideals.[14]

Since women in general are already viewed as lesser than men, various inferiorities are easily attached to women. As many feminist scholars point out, medieval misogynistic views not only minimize women's contributions to economics and politics but also theorize women as lesser beings through theology, philosophy, and science. Women are not simply discriminated against. Discrimination against women is justified through the notion that women are "passive, irrational" and closer to "body, emotion, lust, mercy, and disorder."[15] The polarities that determine women's inferiorities are supported by many different knowledge systems and disciplines.

And this disparity is understood as originating from God's creation. Since the Fall is first caused by Eve, it establishes a scenario in which Eve and all women are bound to their reproductive roles by God's command as punishment. In this view, it is not surprising that women are depicted as craving sex, since by divine will they are supposed to get pregnant and give birth to children.[16]

Seeing women as more physical also leads to other cultural impositions and prejudices. For example, women are often understood as having greater difficulty in achieving the ideal virginal state because of their stronger sexuality.[17] Their craving for sex is evidence that human beings are or became weak due to original sin.[18] The fact that women are weaker than men is also connected to their stronger bodily needs and militated against their ability to achieve the ideal of virginity.

But if childbirth is a punishment, it is also necessary. Since human beings were expelled from paradise and eternal life by taking the forbidden fruit, they must have children to keep humankind going. However, since generation is seen as a substitute for eternal life, coitus is to be initiated only

---

13 Koren, "The Menstruant as 'Other,'" 45.

14 For more implications of masculinity and feminization, see Kruger, "Becoming Christian, Becoming Male?," 21–41.

15 Bynum, "'... And Woman His Humanity,'" 257; Murray, "One Flesh, Two Sexes, Three Genders?," 39.

16 As Karras notes, the medieval concept of female sexuality was different from the Victorian one in that stronger sexual desire was often connected to women in the Middle Ages. Karras, *Sexuality in Medieval Europe*, 56.

17 Karras, *Sexuality in Medieval Europe*, 1.

18 Karras, *Sexuality in Medieval Europe*, 54.

for its proper reason, which is the re-creation of the human form. In other words, sex is acceptable only when a man and a woman have vaginal sex in order to produce a baby. Even when a person feels pleasure during coitus, the delight should not be primary but secondary in that it may help a man or woman produce the semen or fluid needed for a successful pregnancy. Sexual pleasure is legitimate only when it occurs for the sake of offspring. Seeking sexual intercourse only for pleasure is not following God's will.

Women could then be regarded as dangerous in that they are full of more desire than is needed for human generation. As Eve shows in the creation story, women are unable to contain their bodily desires. Eve was defeated by the serpent's temptation and consumed the forbidden fruit, thereby introducing sin into both the bodies and the souls of humankind. In this view, women are created only for reproduction, and it is problematic when they use their sexual nature for anything other than reproductive purposes. Sexual impulses and appetites overflowing from the woman's body are thought of as capable of driving women away from the proper order, and some male theologians are concerned with the danger that women were too licentious to be properly managed. God punishes Eve and controls the evil in her by subjecting her to Adam and limiting her role to propagation. My question is thus: How did women receive these negative characterizations of their bodies, and how did Hildegard of Bingen respond to such depictions?

Purpose of This Book

This book examines porosity as both a physical reality and a theological concept in Hildegard's work. While medieval writers often viewed bodily openness as dangerous—creating risks of contamination, sexual transgression, and moral weakness—Hildegard of Bingen emphasizes its regenerative potential and power. In other words, she uses these concepts of fluidity and porosity to explain women, especially their sexual and reproductive bodies. While representations of the woman's open body appear in different contexts, they all share the ability to receive, hold, and release to the outer world. In a similar sense, Hildegard refers to herself as a trumpet whose tune is played by God.[19] This analogy emphasizes her as an important instrument of God and validates her words as directly coming from God.

---

19 "Sed et loricam fidei induant mites, mansueti, pauperes et miseri existentes, sicut etiam agnus ille fuit, cujus sonus tubae ipsi sunt, mores etiam simplices infantis habentes, quia Deus illos semper flagellat, qui in tuba ipsius canunt, praevidens ne fictile vas illorum pereat, sed ut sibi placcat." Hildegard of Bingen, "Epistola 45," in

This vessel image seems to have helped her survive despite being *magistra* and despite her gender; "[t]he apostle does not permit a woman to teach in Church; but this woman is freed from this condition by the assumption of the Spirit."[20] Her vision offers an alternative understanding: one where the porous female body becomes not a liability but a mirror of the cosmos and a channel of divine vitality. Even God refers to himself as a fountain in Hildegard's vision: "I [God] am Divine Love, the radiance of the living God. Wisdom has done her work with me, and Humility, who is rooted in the living fountain, is my helper...I am the living fountain, because all that was made existed in me like a shadow."[21] Through Hildegard's voice, God emphasizes the vitality of water, presenting himself as both living light and living fountain. Consequently, when women's reproductive bodies inherit God's creative power through their fluidity and porosity, their supposed female weakness transforms into a conduit for new life and healing. The woman's restoration of God's order and reproduction of new life do not occur simply at the individual level but extend to all humankind, parallelling how the Virgin Mary's womb fulfilled its sacred duty of bearing Christ in medieval theological understanding.

Continuing the trajectory of recent studies showing that women navigated their ability and power despite social and religious limitations placed on them, this book highlights how women's physiological difference could become the very source of their spiritual and healing authority. Through close reading of Hildegard's texts, especially her medical treatise and her theological work, I demonstrate how her view of the womb as an instrument of both bodily and spiritual renewal stands out as theologically sophisticated and historically significant. Whether it is in the womb or in God's vessel, the notion of flow is an important one. If menstrual flow stops without proper reasons, it can lead to serious health issues, including infertility. If God's messengers do not deliver God's words to people, it can result in the degeneration of people's devotion and moral behaviour, which Hildegard

---

Hildegard of Bingen, *S. Hildegardis Abbatissae Opera omnia*, col. 217D, as cited in Sur, *Feminine Images of God*, 38.

20 Mews, "Hildegard and the Schools," 109.

21 Hildegard of Bingen, *Book of Divine Works*, trans. Campbell, pt. 3, chap. 3, pp. 387–88. "Ego caritas uiuentis Dei claritas sum, et sapientia mecum opus suum operata est; atquie humilitas, quę in uiuo fonte radicauit, adiutrix mea extitit, . . . Vnde et uiuus fons sum, quia omnia quę facta sunt uelut umbra in me fuerunt" Hildegard of Bingen, *Liber divinorum operum*, ed. Derolez and Dronke, pt. 3, chap. 3, p. 379; Sur, *Feminine Images of God*, 31.

criticizes male priests for. The proper flows not only maintain stable conditions but also heal poor conditions. And the woman's body is represented as a suitable vessel for this flow because it is porous.

Structure of the Book

This book discusses how the woman's body was, and is even now, described and represented as porous and communicative. While the woman's body was often imbued with negative connotations in medieval medicine and theology, this book focuses on Hildegard of Bingen's medical and theological treatises that transformed the woman's body into a place of possibilities for purgation and salvation.

Chapter 1, "Female Porosity and Sacred Flow," establishes how Hildegard of Bingen transformed medieval views of women's bodies from negative to positive. While traditional thought characterized female bodies as dangerously permeable and therefore inferior, Hildegard reinterpreted this porosity as a divine gift enabling purification and spiritual connection. Using the example of Hildegard's own life as a vessel for divine revelation, alongside the theological examples of Eve and Mary, the chapter examines how Hildegard's concept of *viriditas* (greening power) positioned women's physical openness as a strength rather than a weakness. This framework bridges natural science and theology, establishing the foundation for Hildegard's innovative understanding of women's reproductive processes explored throughout the book.

Chapter 2, "The Unsealer of Sin," examines how medieval Christianity understood women's bodies as inherently porous and permeable. While Eve, as the first sinner, introduced sin and death to humankind through her vulnerability, the Virgin Mary's receptive womb brought salvation by bearing the Saviour. These contrasting female figures provided Hildegard of Bingen with rich conceptual frameworks for theorizing the female body, allowing her to bridge natural science and theology. This chapter also introduces Hildegard's life and works, particularly her self-understanding as a divine messenger transmitting God's words to humanity. As a communicator between sacred and worldly realms, Hildegard emphasized women's mediating position in both reproduction and salvation.

Chapter 3, "Releasing Blood and Humours," investigates women's reproductive processes, which medieval thought attributed to the physical openness of the female body. Unlike many of her contemporaries, who viewed menstruation and female sexuality negatively, Hildegard presents a more nuanced understanding of women's embodied experiences, highlighting how these processes serve important purgative functions. Hildegard's categorization of women by temperament further challenges medieval stereotypes by acknowledging women's physiological diversity.

Chapter 4, "Receiving the Spirit, Foam, and Fluids," develops the concept of female porosity to explore women's life-giving capabilities in both biological reproduction and spiritual salvation. Hildegard's understanding of conception emphasizes complementary male and female contributions, with the woman's body actively purifying, warming, and transforming the male seed. This chapter examines how Hildegard connects these physical processes to spiritual concepts, particularly through her notion of *viriditas*.

Chapter 5, "Giving Birth to a Baby and Giving Spiritual Birth to Humankind," elaborates on how Hildegard conceptualizes holy flows through women's bodies. The chapter analyzes Hildegard's vision of Ecclesia as a female figure whose perforated womb receives and purifies souls, drawing parallels between physical childbirth and spiritual salvation. For Hildegard, the female body's capacity for flow becomes a powerful metaphor for divine redemption.

While the chapters in the body of the book focus on medieval European contexts, the afterword widens the scope by analysing Korean folk medicine practices that similarly utilize concepts of the porosity of female reproductive organs, suggesting cross-cultural continuities in understanding women's bodies as sites of both vulnerability and power.

Throughout the book, the terms "porosity" and "flow" are central to analysing Hildegard's depiction of women's reproductive and spiritual bodies. "Porosity," in this context, refers specifically to the physical and symbolic openness and permeability of the woman's body—especially evident in reproductive functions like menstruation, conception, and childbirth—which Hildegard reinterprets from a traditionally negative vulnerability into a positive, salvational quality. Similarly, the notion of "flow" encapsulates not merely physical fluids (such as blood, humours, and milk) but also the dynamic movement of spiritual energy, grace, and salvation through the female body. Together, these concepts illuminate how Hildegard transforms the medieval understanding of the female body from passive receptivity into active engagement with divine and natural processes. Each chapter will reinforce and clarify how Hildegard applies and redefines these terms, ultimately revealing their integrative role in her theological and medical visions. This framework allows us to see how Hildegard's innovative approach challenges conventional medieval theological and medical understandings of the female body, repositioning women's reproductive capacities as central rather than peripheral to salvation history.

Chapter 1

FEMALE POROSITY AND SACRED FLOW

FROM EVE AND MARY TO HILDEGARD OF BINGEN

HILDEGARD OF BINGEN was an extraordinary figure whose life embodied the very porosity that she attributed to the female body in her medical and theological works.[1] Born into a noble family in 1098, she was dedicated to the Church as the age of eight as a tithe to God—the tenth and last child of her parents. This early surrender made her physically and spiritually permeable to divine influence from a young age. She claimed to have experienced visions since early childhood, though she initially kept these experiences hidden. As she later wrote, "From my earliest childhood, before my bones, nerves, and veins were fully strengthened, I have always seen this vision in my soul, even to the present time when I am more than seventy years old."[2] Although she started to publicly share her receipt of visions when she was in her forties, her hagiography asserts that she was so open to visions from God that she even received visions before being born.[3] In other words, she was open to God's messages even in her mother's womb.

Hildegard was sent to live with Jutta of Sponheim, a female hermit, at the age of eight, and they entered an enclosure belonging to the Benedictine monastery of Disibodenberg with two other women on November 1, 1112. Under Jutta's guidance, Hildegard learned to read Scripture, particularly the Psalms, in Latin. Despite her claims of being "unlearned" and "simple," Hildegard clearly received a substantial education. After Jutta's death in 1136, Hildegard became *magistra*, mother, and abbess to the women at Disibodenberg while her community was growing. In this transitional role, Hildegard's first significant act of spiritual and physical boundary-crossing appeared, which would then continue throughout her life.

In 1141, at the age of forty-two, Hildegard had a pivotal mystical experience that transformed her relationship to her visions. She described this moment as one of profound physical permeability: "Heaven was opened

---

1 For more information about her life and its sources, see Embach, "The Life of Hildegard of Bingen," 11–36.

2 *Vita Sanctae Hildegardis*, ed. Klaes, 3.

3 Newman, "Hildegard and Her Hagiographers," 19.

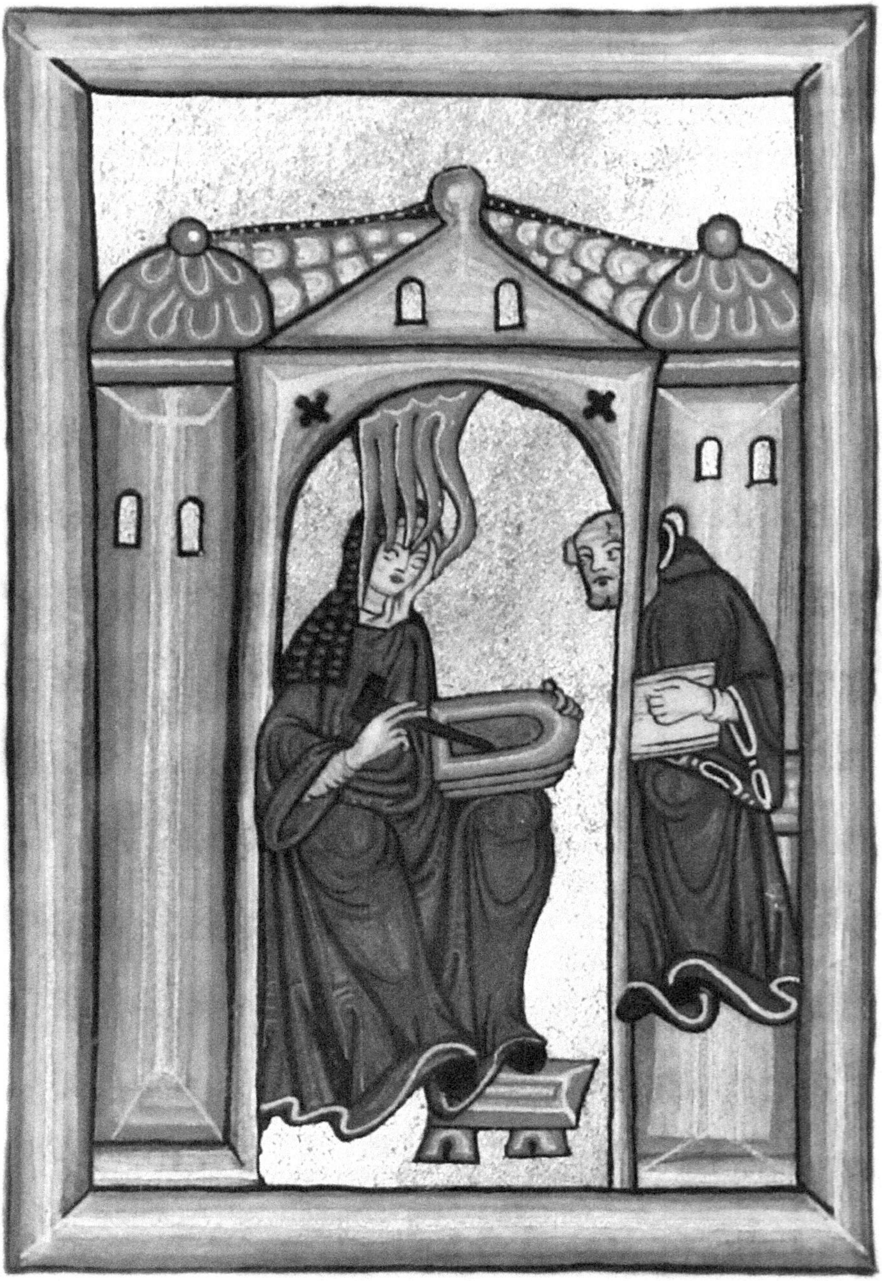

Figure 1. "Hildegard with Flaming Light of Fire."
In Hildegard of Bingen, *Scivias Codex*, pt. 1, vision 1, fol. 1r, ca. 1175.
Original lost, hand-copied on parchment, ca. 1930. Rüdesheim-Eibingen, St. Hildegard's Abbey. Courtesy of St. Hildegard's Abbey.

and a fiery light of exceeding brilliance came and permeated my whole brain, and inflamed my whole heart and my whole breast, not like a burning but like a warming flame."[4] This divine illumination and word literally flowed through her bodily boundaries, entering not just her mind but her heart and breast as well. In her portrait along with her secretary Volmar in the manuscript of *Scivias*, she is receiving a flame directly to her head, observed by Volmar.

According to Margot Fassler, this portrait is unique, with imagery not seen in other authors' portraits.[5] And the illustrations that depicts her writing all share a presentation of her as porous and therefore a vessel of God's visual and verbal messages. Her own emphasis on being "uneducated," although it seems that it was a part of her humility *topos*, has the effect of making her the vessel of God's messages. The notion that religious women served as "vessels" for God was often accompanied by a *topos* that women ultimately had no choice but to let the words of God pour out from them. Hildegard repeatedly insisted that she was so uneducated that there was no way she could have just been pretending her knowledge originated from God, something that can be also found in the lives of other female saints in the Middle Ages. It meant that she should be open to receive and at the same time to spit out God's words.

After receiving a divine command to "[s]ay and write what you see and hear," Hildegard initially hesitated to follow this instruction. Her reluctance was overcome when her body manifested her spiritual struggle,[6] something that can be found in the experience of other mystical women such as Angela of Foligno and Catherine of Siena. This pattern, using bodily illness to communicate divine displeasure, became a significant strategy in Hildegard's life, demonstrating how her physical body functioned as a medium between earthly and divine realms. With Bernard of Clairvaux's help, Hildegard received permission from Pope Eugenius III to record her

---

4 Hildegard of Bingen, *Scivias*, trans. Hart and Bishop, 59. "Maximae coruscationis igneum lumen aperto caelo ueniens totum cerebrum meum transfudit et totum cor totumque pectus meum uelut flamma non tamen ardens sed calens ita inflammauit." Hildegard of Bingen, "Protestificatio veracium visionum a deo fluentium," *Scivias*, ed. Führkötter and Carelvaris, 3–4.

5 Fassler, *Cosmos, Liturgy, and the Arts*, 67.

6 "In the meantime, because I have kept silent about this vision, I have been laid low, bedridden in my infirmities, and am unable to raise myself up." "Hildegard to Bernard, Abbot of Clairvaux," in Hildegard of Bingen, *Letters*, trans. Baird and Ehrman, no. 1, 1:28.

visions.[7] This papal approval allowed her to cross the gendered boundary that typically prevented women from working as teachers or theologians. Her body became a channel for divine knowledge, enabling her to transcend the normal limitations placed on women in the medieval Church. In a letter to her spiritual companion Elizabeth of Schönau, Hildegard described this sacred permeability that she performed throughout her life: "Human being is a vessel, which God built for himself, and which he imbued with his breath, so that he might complete his works in it."[8]

Perhaps the most dramatic example of Hildegard's bodily porosity as a strategic tool came when she decided to move her community from Disibodenberg to Rupertsberg. When the abbot resisted her plan, Hildegard fell ill, interpreting her sickness as divine punishment for her failure to fulfil God's will, similar to her sickness when she refused to write down her visions. Eventually, her strategic "charismatic illness" convinced the Church authorities to withdraw their objections, allowing her to establish an independent female community at Rupertsberg.[9] Later, she founded a second community at Eibingen, further demonstrating her remarkable ability to cross established boundaries through her claimed divine connection to her body.

Her connections reached to people, too. During her life, Hildegard of Bingen maintained a lively correspondence with the powerful figures of her time, including emperors, popes, and theologians. Her letters show her moving fluidly between the postures of humility and authority—describing herself as a "poor little weak form of a woman"[10] while simultaneously delivering bold prophetic admonitions to male authorities who had "the twin advantages of formal education and gender superiority in a patriarchal society."[11] This rhetorical fluidity allowed her to speak with authority while acknowledging the gendered limitations of her position.

Hildegard's intellectual output demonstrates a similarly permeable quality. She moved between genres and disciplines with remarkable facility, producing works of theology based on her visions, such as *Scivias*, the *Liber vitae meritorum*, and the *Liber divinorum operum*; natural science and

---

7 Feiss, "Introduction," 13.

8 Rapp, "A Woman Speaks," 21.

9 Newman, "Introduction," 13.

10 "Hildegard to the Monks," in Hildegard of Bingen, *Letters*, trans. Baird and Ehrman, no. 113r, 2:59.

11 Kerby-Fulton, "Prophet and Reformer," 72.

medicine, such as *Cause et cure* and *Physica*; music, such as the *Symphonia*; hagiography; and even an invented language. Her theological and medical works, in particular, represent how she understood the female body as not merely a passive vessel but an active participant in creation, healing, and spiritual transformation.

Hildegard's self-representation as a vessel of God's knowledge worked well in two ways. First, it helped her build authority as a female religious figure, permitting her to channel divine wisdom without claiming personal credit. Second, it enabled her to redefine the vessel image itself, transforming it from a symbol of passivity to one of active mediation, which was not limited to her individual case but extended to all women. Just as she depicted the woman's womb as actively purifying male semen during conception, as will be discussed further later, Hildegard presented herself as actively processing and communicating divine knowledge.

Hildegard died on September 17, 1179, having lived until the remarkable age of eighty-one. Despite popular veneration during her life, she was not officially canonized until 2012, when she was also named a Doctor of the Church—one of only four women to be formally recognized as contributing to the Church intellectually.[12] Granted that the canonization process is complicated and easily influenced by social and political circumstances, Hildegard's delayed official recognition reflects the complex position she occupied as a woman who frequently transcended the boundaries placed upon her sex, remaining, like her view of the female body itself, too fluid to be easily contained or fixed by ecclesiastical categories.

Theorizing Female Porosity: Historical Continuity

Hildegard of Bingen did not invent the concept of female porosity. The understanding of women's bodies as fundamentally porous has deep historical roots, extending from ancient Greek medical theories through medieval theology and into modern scholarly analysis. The humoral theories that informed Hildegard's understanding of the woman's body represent not a medieval discovery but rather the inheritance of ancient Greco-Roman medico-philosophical traditions that continued to evolve for centuries before and after her death. These concepts of female porosity, both as physiological reality and as spiritual metaphor, demonstrate remarkable persistence

---

12 The other female Doctors of the Church are Angela of Foligno, Catherine of Siena, and Teresa of Ávila.

across disparate historical contexts. What distinguishes Hildegard is not that she rejected these inherited ideas about women's permeable bodies, but rather that she reinterpreted them through her unique theological vision, transforming potential liabilities into spiritual assets.

Numerous historians and philosophers have uncovered this persistent thread in Western thinking about gender and embodiment. Scholars such as Thomas Laqueur, Joan Cadden, and Monica Green have demonstrated how Galenic and Aristotelian models positioned the female body as inherently more open, moist, and permeable than its male counterpart.[13] These physiological theories found profound expression in medieval religious and literary contexts. Modern feminist scholarship has further illuminated how concepts of female porosity shaped gendered power dynamics. In particular, the work of Caroline Walker Bynum on religious women's bodily practices reveals how medieval Christian culture understood female physicality through its capacity for transformation and permeability.[14] The porous female body was also believed to create vulnerability that made women more easily possessed by either God or evil spirits.[15]

Leah DeVun has analyzed how women were linked to softness and leakage, demonstrating how this feminine porosity became equated with moral weakness, "which might invite feminine vanity, torpor, and decadence" and potentially corrupt manly men and the entire social order in the High Middle Ages.[16] DeVun points out that medieval authorities located women's sexuality specifically in the body's openings and pathways, citing how Isidore traced female desire to the umbilicus, while other authorities attributed it to "an anatomically open pathway to the uterus."[17] Such anatomical explanations reinforced the association between female openness and moral vulnerability.

Building on this historical view of female porosity, Vern Bullough demonstrates that misogynistic attitudes towards women's bodies were not solely religious in origin but deeply rooted in ancient medical traditions that medieval scholars inherited.[18] Bullough shows how Aristotelian notions posi-

13 Laqueur, *Making Sex*; Cadden, *Meanings of Sex Difference*; Green, *Making Women's Medicine Masculine.*

14 Bynum, *Holy Feast and Holy Fast.*

15 Caciola, *Discerning Spirits.*

16 DeVun, "Erecting Sex," 29.

17 DeVun, "Erecting Sex," 30.

18 Bullough, "Marriage in the Middle Ages," 485–501.

tioning women as "incomplete men" with inherently inferior, porous bodies were seamlessly integrated into medieval thought systems, even appearing in the works of prominent theologians like Thomas Aquinas. These classical medical traditions, particularly Galen's characterization of women as colder, moister, and fundamentally more permeable versions of the male ideal, provided seemingly scientific justification for women's subordination. The persistence of these medical theories about female porosity—that women's bodies were intrinsically more open, leaky, and susceptible to external influences—offered learned authorities a "natural" explanation for restricting women's roles and mobility, one that operated alongside and often reinforced religious restrictions.

Similarly, feminist philosophers have examined how feminine fluidity challenges dominant patriarchal discourse. This concept of female fluidity has attracted significant attention from feminist scholars, particularly those employing psychoanalytic approaches. For these theorists, the metaphors of women's instability and flow provide frameworks for understanding both historical oppression and potential resistance. In *Speculum of the Other Woman*, for instance, Luce Irigaray further develops this concept through her critique of the mechanics of solids that has dominated Western thought. She contrasts this with a mechanics of fluids that better represents feminine experience. Women are not fixed but constantly changing—neither open nor closed. "This incompleteness in her form, her morphology, allows her continually to become something else, though this is not to say that she is ever univocally nothing."[19] While the flowing and fluid are referred to as "shameful," "deforming," and "abhorrent" by men,[20] this fluid discourse reflects the physical reality of female bodies that flow monthly, that change shape during pregnancy, that emit milk—all processes that Hildegard, centuries earlier, had recognized as divinely ordained rather than deficient.

While the woman's womb was the place of human origins, it was often compared to the enclosed garden. Liz McAvoy extensively explores how garden imagery, particularly the enclosed garden, reinforces the paradoxical nature of the female body, both open and closed, both dangerous and sacred, that appears consistently throughout medieval writing about women. Through religious and literary texts, she demonstrates how the female body functioned simultaneously as theological metaphor and physical reality, its permeability serving various symbolic and practical purposes in religious

19 Irigaray, *Speculum of the Other Woman*, 229.

20 Irigaray, *Speculum of the Other Woman*, 237.

discourse. Women's logic of flux is contrasted to the "monolithic, fixed, phallic" reasoning of men, establishing a gender binary based fundamentally on concepts of containment and flow.[21] Also, McAvoy points out, "these 'feminine' drives based on fluidity, change and renewal tend to become focused upon desire, natality and the maternal, and, like the unconscious, erupt periodically into the text via lacunae in the latter to offer challenge to the intransigence of the Law."[22] Thus, women's supposed instability becomes reframed as a potential weapon against the male-centred Church and society. Women's fluid nature can have transformative power.

McAvoy introduces many medieval writings on this subject, and interpretations by feminists who have adapted psychoanalytic approaches to understand medieval women's mystical and physical experience also emphasize women's state of constant movement as "efflorescence."[23] As McAvoy rightly points out, the close association between the woman's body and the garden repeatedly emphasizes female porosity in medieval thought. The enclosed garden, *hortus conclusus*, which appears prominently in the *Song of Songs* and its exegeses as well as in Marian adoration, represents the paradoxical nature of the virginal woman's body, which is simultaneously closed to worldly corruption yet open to divine influence. These gardens are explicitly described as "closed and sealed" against improper entry; yet, crucially, they remain permeable to the right influences, allowing them to flourish, create, and reproduce.[24] This imagery perfectly captures the medieval ambivalence toward female porosity: a quality that required careful containment yet remained essential for fulfilling divine purposes.

In this regard, the virginal body presents a fascinating paradox in medieval thought. The Virgin Mary's body is traditionally portrayed as sealed—the quintessential enclosed vessel. Laura Miles examines medieval interpretations of the Annunciation scene to highlight this enclosed nature of Mary's body. Yet her body cannot be entirely sealed, as her womb both receives and delivers God. As Miles notes, in Goscelin of St. Bertin's *Liber confortatorius*, "the Lord would be watching over his 'going in,' in his conception, and over his 'going out,' in his birth."[25] This tension between closure and openness

21 McAvoy, *The Enclosed Garden*, 85.

22 McAvoy, *The Enclosed Garden*, 85.

23 McAvoy, *The Enclosed Garden*, 29.

24 McAvoy, *The Enclosed Garden*, 35.

25 Barnes et al., *Writing the Wilton Women*, 166; Miles, *The Virgin Mary's Book*, 55–57.

creates a productive theological ambiguity that medieval thinkers like Hildegard would explore.

Even much later, in eighteenth-century Germany, Barbara Duden identifies "clear echoes and yet fleeting shadows of ideas about humours, fluxes, and the openness of the flesh" of women in medical writings that originated in archaic Greek tradition.[26] This remarkable continuity demonstrates how deeply entrenched these concepts were in Western medical and cultural thought. Similarly, Hildegard's work reveals these ancient concepts not merely as medical theories but as living traditions that shaped both practical medicine and theological understanding in the Middle Ages. However, as DeVun, Bullough, McAvoy, Miles, Duden, and many others demonstrate, "the history of the sexes is a history of the contingent, the changing, and therefore the changeable."[27] It is precisely this changeability that Hildegard seizes upon, transforming traditional notions of female porosity into a positive theological vision.

And this porosity, although it will be fully discussed in later chapters of this book, is very vividly represented in Hildegard's concept of *viriditas*, the generative greening power essential to creation. Central to Hildegard's reconceptualization of female porosity was her distinctive understanding of this greening power. While the term had precedent in theological writings—Augustine and Gregory both used it to describe spiritual vitality—Hildegard radically expanded its application to encompass physical processes, particularly those of the female body.[28] For her, *viriditas* represented not merely spiritual vigour but the divine life-force manifest in all creation, flowing most visibly in women's bodies through menstruation, pregnancy, and childbirth. This conceptual innovation allowed her to transform traditional understandings of female "leakiness" from a liability into a privileged connection to divine creative power.

Where her contemporaries saw female fluidity primarily as a danger requiring containment, Hildegard recognized in it a reflection of divine creative power—a means through which the redemptive "greening" of humanity could occur.[29] In her book on Hildegard's medical knowledge, Sweet has pointed out the central importance of fluidity in Hildegard's *Cause et cure*, particularly how Hildegard's positive depiction of the female body is

---

26 Duden, *The Woman Beneath the Skin*, 33.

27 DeVun, "Erecting Sex," 37.

28 Sweet, *Rooted in the Earth*, 140–42.

29 Fassler, *Cosmos, Liturgy, and the Arts*, 209, 233.

intrinsically linked to her concept of *viriditas*. Sweet suggests that Hildegard would have been exposed to the concept of *viriditas* in the writings of the Church Fathers who adapted this word to signify the growth of good qualities such as faith or love, based on plants' fertility and greenness.[30] However, Sweet also points out that Hildegard's usage of *viriditas* is unique in using this concept beyond botanical and theological studies.[31] Hildegard expanded the concept of *viriditas* to encompass human physiology, asserting that the body itself possesses this greening power, with the female body in particular embodying this creative force.

Hildegard interprets *viriditas* as flowing power, causing the flow of humours, blood, and moisture so that the body can function in the right way. It grows the bodily members of the foetus. It is something that grows hair on one's head or chin. At the same time, moisture is much needed in Hildegard's gynaecology and can be carried by the help of *viriditas*. Throughout her medical and theological works, Hildegard establishes a direct correlation between women's menstrual cycles and the concept of *viriditas*.

> The stream of a woman's menstrual period is her life-giving *viriditas*[32] and her exuberant vigor. This sprouts into offspring, as a tree with its vital force sprouts and flowers, producing leaves and fruits. So a woman, from the vital force of the menstrual blood, produces flowers and leaves in the fruit of her womb.[33]

Hildegard's *viriditas* is directly related to flowing and flowering. For example, Hildegard explains that infertility in younger and older women is caused directly by their physiological deficiency in *viriditas*—a condition that she

---

30 Sweet, *Rooted in the Earth*, 141–42.

31 Sweet, *Rooted in the Earth*, 150–54.

32 In analysing Hildegard's complex terminology, I have deliberately preserved the Latin *viriditas* rather than adopting Throop's translation of "vital force." This philological decision maintains the term's multivalent significance within Hildegard's corpus, encompassing connotations of verdant fecundity, vital essence, and generative plenitude that operate simultaneously across her natural philosophy, gynaecological writings, and horticultural observations. The untranslated term better preserves the conceptual intersection between theological vitality and biological generativity central to Hildegard's integrated cosmology.

33 Hildegard of Bingen, *Causes and Cures*, trans. Throop, 87. "Riuulus autem menstrui temporis in muliere est genitiua uiriditas et floriditas eius, que in prole frondet, quia ut arbor uiriditate sua floret et frondet et fructus profert, sic femina de uiriditate riuulorum menstrui sanguinis flores et frondes in fructu uentris sui educit." Hildegard of Bingen, *Beate Hildegardis Cause et cure*, ed. Moulinier and Berndt, bk. 2, §227, p. 145.

explicitly parallels with arboreal biology, wherein trees lacking sufficient sap (their botanical *viriditas*) fail to generate flowers and fruit from their roots. This botanical–gynaecological homology exemplifies Hildegard's emphasis on flowing as an integrated natural philosophy.

At the same time, this physiological function is presented not as mere biological necessity or fertility. For Hildegard, *viriditas* was also the embodiment of divine creative force, positioning the female body as a vessel of sacred generative capacity within the medieval cosmological framework, highlighting female porosity in spiritual and physical senses. Occasionally, Hildegard uses this greening power in relation to the soul when she discusses the soul's ability to send the vital power of *viriditas* so that the soul can grow or maintain the bodily members.

> I [soul] am the living breath in a human being, placed in a tabernacle of marrow, veins, bones and flesh, giving it vitality [*viriditas*] and supporting its every movement.[34]

> ...for it gives vitality [*viriditas*] to the marrow and veins and members of the whole body, as the tree from its root gives sap and greenness [*viriditas*] to all the branches.[35]

This *viriditas*, the greening power, is closely connected to the *vivens fons*, or "living fountain" in English, and the Garden of Eden where the first human beings were placed. Furthermore, Hildegard uses water images in association with *viriditas* in emphasizing its power to grow trees, in contrast to dryness and desiccation.[36] Hildegard emphasized this vital greenness in her music as well and indicated that this vital greening power must ultimately be restored through salvation, returning eternal verdancy to humanity. In her illuminated manuscripts, Hildegard frequently depicted *viriditas* as streams of moisture flowing between divine and human realms, often col-

---

34 Hildegard of Bingen, *Scivias*, trans. Hart and Bishop, 113. "Spiraculum tamen uiuens in homine sum, posita in tabernaculum medullarum, uenarum, ossium et carnis, ita quod eidem tabernaculo uiriditatem tribuo et quod illud ubique in motibus suis circumfero." Hildegard of Bingen, *Scivias*, ed. Führkötter and Carelvaris, pt. 1, bk. 4, chap. 4, p. 67.

35 In the English version, *viriditas* was translated as "vitality" and "greenness" in this sentence. Hildegard of Bingen, *Scivias*, trans. Hart and Bishop, 120. "Quoniam uiriditatem medullarum ac uenarum et omnium membrorum toti corpori tribuit, uelut arbor ex sua radice sucum et uiriditatem omnibus ramis dat." Hildegard of Bingen, *Scivias*, ed. Führkötter and Carelvaris, pt. 1, bk. 4, chap. 16, p. 78.

36 Peter Loewen argues that Hildegard of Bingen followed the Church Fathers' use of the concept of greenness, especially Gregory's understanding of *viriditas* in spiritual terms. See Loewen, "From the Root to the Branches," 125–69.

oured green to emphasize its connection to growth and fertility. This visual language reinforced her understanding that female bodily processes participate in cosmic patterns of flow rather than representing dangerous aberrations requiring containment. By associating women's physiological processes with this sacred moisture, the same divine moisture that greens the earth after rain and sustains all living things, Hildegard created a theological framework that dignified female embodiment. As we will see, this concept became the cornerstone of her positive reinterpretation of menstruation, conception, and childbirth as sacred rather than polluting processes.

Menstruation and the Porosity of Women's Bodies

Menstruation is the most visible example of a woman's porous body with flow in and out, and medieval medicine acknowledges the importance of menstruation. Many medieval books claim that menstruation is needed not only for conception but also for general health. Menstruation is assumed to be necessary for a woman's body because it does not have the same qualities as a man's body. The female body is so lacking in heat and dryness that it has to expel its waste regularly. Because menstruation is seen as the residue of waste, it is understood as polluting, a notion that is not new in the Middle Ages. The toxic nature of menstruation can be traced all the way back to ancient Greek medicine and natural science. In the physical and medical view of medieval Christianity, women's reproductive organs and their processes are understood as permeable in ways that are both necessary and potentially toxic.

This notion of menstruation as pollution is easily seen in the book *De secretis mulierum*, "Regarding Women's Secrets" in English, composed in the thirteenth or early fourteenth century and falsely attributed to Albertus Magnus, although it is not just Pseudo-Albertus Magnus who believes in poisonous menstruation.[37] As Green comments, this book is "one of the most influential documents in the history of medieval scientific attitudes toward women."[38] While the superficial purpose of the book is to instruct the reader

37 This manuscript contains a mix of voices—the author (possibly Pseudo-Albertus Magnus), Commentary A, and Commentary B. While the English translation and its Latin manuscript reference combine these different sources, I have not distinguished between them in my analysis.

38 According to Green, this book was neither the first nor the last work to be entitled "women's secrets." From the middle of the thirteenth century, texts began to be written under this title with the common goal of letting men in on the hidden secrets

in biological facts about human generation, the authors repeatedly emphasize women's polluting and dangerous sexuality. The real aim of *De secretis mulierum* is thus to convince men of women's evil and dangerous nature, and in so doing, make them warier of women's sexual bodies.[39]

According to Pseudo-Albertus, women often cause harm even when they do not intend to because of the polluting nature of their bodies. The evidence for this notion, as Pseudo-Albertus presents it, lies in women's menstruation. He explains menstruation according to the medieval medical understanding of it as a monthly purgation of excess food.[40] However, menstrual blood is not merely residual food: it is much more toxic and harmful than dietary waste alone would be.[41] In order to show that women's menses are like venom, Pseudo-Albertus draws not only on ancient medical theory but also on popular belief, arguing, for example, that if any tree was touched by menstrual fluid, it would immediately lose its vitality.[42] Also, if babies in cradles are stared at by menstruating women, it would harm them.[43]

Possible effects of this "venom" in women's menstrual fluid also include a predisposition for epilepsy and leprosy in children conceived during menstruation. When Pseudo-Albertus advises men not to have intercourse with

---

supposed to exist regarding women's sexual and reproductive bodies. Green, "From 'Diseases of Women' to 'Secrets of Women,'" 14–15. The work has 105 surviving copies; in particular, it seems that it enjoyed great popularity in the fifteenth century insofar as three-fourths of the surviving copies were produced in this period. Green appreciated how quickly this book appeared in print and how rapidly it spread, considering the fact that printed versions of it started to appear by 1475. Green, *Making Women's Medicine Masculine*, 212n31.

39 Lemay, "Introduction," 16.

40 Pseudo-Albertus Magnus, *Women's Secrets*, trans. Lemay, 69. Lemay primarily relied on the Lyons 1590 edition for this translation. "Iuxta quod notandum quod menstruum in muliere nichil aliud est quam superfluum alimenti quod in substanciam rei alende non cedit, sicut est in viris sperma. Et vocatur 'menstruum' in muliere quia fluit quolibet mense ad minus semel cum mulier tante etatis fuerit, hoc est, novem annorum, ut frequencius accidit. Tunc incipit esse fluxus menstruorum quolibet mense propter nature purgacionem." Pseudo-Albertus Magnus, *El "De secretis mulierum,"* trans. Barragán Nieto, chap. 1, §§31–37, pp. 234–36.

41 Pseudo-Albertus Magnus, *El "De secretis mulierum,"* trans. Barragán Nieto, chap. 1, §§49–53, p. 238.

42 This excerpt from Commentary B is absent from the Lyons 1590 edition of the text. Commentary B represents a separate gloss tradition not included in this particular manuscript. Pseudo-Albertus Magnus, *Women's Secrets*, trans. Lemay, 75.

43 Pseudo-Albertus Magnus, *Women's Secrets*, trans. Lemay, 129. Pseudo-Albertus Magnus, *El "De secretis mulierum,"* trans. Barragán Nieto, chap. 8, §§30–34, p. 450.

women during their period (after providing tips for recognizing whether a woman is menstruating or not), he offers the cautionary information that epilepsy and leprosy would be caused by toxic menstruation.[44] The idea that intercourse with a woman during her period could cause leprosy was a widely held belief. Yet women were not affected by their venomous menses as long as they did not retain them. On the other hand, menstrual fluids could always potentially harm men and animals, even at a distance.[45] The implied danger of women's sexual fluids also sometimes occasioned another belief in the toxicity of women's bodies. Some people suggest that certain women are fine even after they swallow poisonous materials,[46] which in turn helps to explain why women are protected from their own poison even if their menstrual fluids are toxic to men.[47]

On the other hand, women can also become sick if they do not menstruate. According to the cultural belief that menstruation is pollution, if they experience menstruation retention, the toxins in their menses will accumulate. Apparently, however, sexual activity can help them avoid such accumulation. This sickness happens in women because they are full of corrupt and poisonous menses, and therefore it is good that these women, whether young or old, often use men, so that this matter might be expelled. This is especially helpful in young women because they are full of humidity.[48] Thus,

---

44 Pseudo-Albertus Magnus, *Women's Secrets*, trans. Lemay, 129. "Et caveat sibi quivis quod tunc non coeat, quia pueri qui in menstruis fluentibus concipiuntur maiorem inclinacionem habent ad morbum caducum et ad lepram. Et tales huiusmodi infirmitates qua alia cicius inficiuntur lepra, quare propter talem venenositatem mulierum nocivum est coire." Pseudo-Albertus Magnus. *El "De secretis mulierum,"* trans. Barragán Nieto, chap. 8, §§27–28, p. 448n.

45 Pseudo-Albertus Magnus, *Women's Secrets*, trans. Lemay, 60. In this footnote, I reference a different edition for the Latin text, since it includes essential commentary absent in the critical edition. The following is from Commentary A. "Et hoc ideo quia mulieres sunt tempore menstrui venenose, ita quòd intoxicant animalia per visum, inficiunt pueros in cunis, maculant speculum bene tersum, et quandoque faciunt coeuntem cum ipsis leprosum fieri, quandoque cancrosum. Et quia malum non euitatur nisi cognitum, ideò necesse est vulentibus abstiner cognoscere immunditiam coius, et multa alia qua in hoc libro docetur, et sic Albertus videns quod iustè peteret, consensit ei, et sic tangitur causa effeciès, mota cùm dicitur scribo, et sic." "Prooemium" in Pseudo-Albertus Magnus, *De secretis mulierum*, 5–6.

46 Jacquart and Thomasset, *Sexuality and Medicine*, 92.

47 Jacquart and Thomasset, *Sexuality and Medicine*, 191.

48 Pseudo-Albertus Magnus, *Women's Secrets*, trans. Lemay, 132. "Hec autem egritudo contingit mulieribus quia multum habundat in eis de menstruo quod corruptum est et venenosum. Et ideo cautum est et bonum ut tales, quecumque fuerint sive

menstrual blood or menses can lead to sickness or madness in women who try to lead an ascetic life because they do not have the chance to eliminate their bodily toxins through sexual activity.[49]

These ideas must have been enough to drive home a negative image of the female body to male readers, as they reinforce a pervasive phobia of women's hidden reproductive anatomy and their dangerous bodily fluids. While Pseudo-Albertus's book was popular among medieval men, other male writers also accept the toxicity of menstruation and the polluting nature of menstruating women.

Hildegard's Porosity of Women and the Whole World

But are only women porous? For Hildegard, human beings' sin made not only their own bodies but also the whole world porous, too. Once humankind fell from its pure and perfect state, the offspring of Adam and Eve were impacted by the aftermath, becoming porous and adaptable to change to survive in their degenerated state. Once the first human beings became open to the original sin, they were all exposed to the need to purge themselves on a regular basis. Women have a more regular process for purging themselves: menstruation. However, men also have their own ways to cleanse themselves through sweat, although they were believed to have greater heat and did not need to have regular bleeding.

And according to Hildegard's micro-macrocosm, the whole world had also degenerated from its original state since the first human beings. Before Adam's transgression, the world was not movable and did not need to move, as it was perfect as it was. However, once the human body became imperfect and needed purgation, the whole cosmos succumbed to the same destiny, needing to be cleansed on a regular basis.

> Before the fall of Adam, the firmament was immobile and did not revolve; after his fall, it began to move and revolve; after the last day, it will stand immobile, as in the first creation, before Adam's fall. Now, however, it revolves, and is strengthened and firmed by the sun, moon, and stars. If it stood motionless, it would quickly flow away, having become liquid and soft.[50]

---

iuvenes sive antique, sepe viris utantur, ut materia talis expellatur. Iuvenibus autem multum expedit que in humido habundant." Pseudo-Albertus Magnus, *El "De secretis mulierum,"* trans. Barragán Nieto, chap. 9, §§22–27, p. 460.

49 Jacquart and Thomasset, *Sexuality and Medicine*, 174.

50 Hildegard of Bingen, *Causes and Cures*, trans. Throop, 9. "Ante casum Ade firmamentum immobile fuit et non circumuoluebatur, post casum autem eius cepit moueri et circumuolui; sed post nouissimum diem inmobile stabit, ut in prima creatione ante

Previously, the firmament did not move and did not need to move.[51] However, Adam's transgression made it move. According to Hildegard's view, it seems that the whole cosmos, including the heavens, started to suffer from venoms and poisons. Therefore, its motion works as a useful way to purge these poisons when the firmament is not in the purest state. The moving and revolving state is now required, and the firmament would have problems without it.

> If it [the firmament] stood motionless, it would quickly flow away, having become liquid and soft. Because it revolves, it cleanses the elements. This cleansing sometimes consists of visible watery, dark clouds; just as water, placed in a pot on the fire, throws off a foam in the boiling heat, and is cleansed.[52]

For Hildegard, in this degenerated cosmos, the firmament should keep moving. Its movement allows the firmament to clean itself through "visible watery, dark clouds." For Hildegard, the dark colour signifies the negativity.

Hildegard also utilizes the imagery of a pot during this cleansing process. In the later parts of this book, I revisit Hildegard's concept of a vessel or pot to highlight porosity in her optimistic cosmology and anthropology. While vessel or pot images have been popularly used to explain the female body that menstruates and gives birth through an association with weakness, here it is the firmament that becomes weakened; yet, precisely due to this weakness, it achieves self-purification.

---

casum Ade fuit. Nunc autem ideo circumuoluitur, ut a sole, luna et stellis roboretur et confirmetur, quia si inmobile staret, cito liquefactum et emollitum deflueret." Hildegard of Bingen, *Beate Hildegardis Cause et cure*, ed. Moulinier and Berndt, bk. 1, §27, p. 32.

51 The firmament was characterized as a luminous, tenuous expanse, frequently connected with celestial radiance. This characterization corresponds to exegetical traditions emphasizing its ethereal qualities, particularly evident in the Songs of the Sabbath Sacrifice, where textual evidence associates it with the radiance of angelic vestments. Within ancient cosmological frameworks, the firmament constituted one element in a restricted cosmographic taxonomy, typically juxtaposed with heaven and the primordial waters, signifying its function as a fundamental structural component in premodern cosmic architecture.

52 Hildegard of Bingen, *Causes and Cures*, trans. Throop, 9. "Quia si inmobile staret, cito liquefactum et emollitum deflueret. Ex hoc etiam, quod modo circumuoluitur, elementa purgat, et purgatio illa interdum sunt aquose et nigre nubes, quas uidemus, uelut etiam aqua, cum ad ignem in olla ponitur, et in feruore caloris spumam eicit et purgatur." Hildegard of Bingen, *Beate Hildegardis Cause et cure*, ed. Moulinier and Berndt, bk. 1, §27, p. 32.

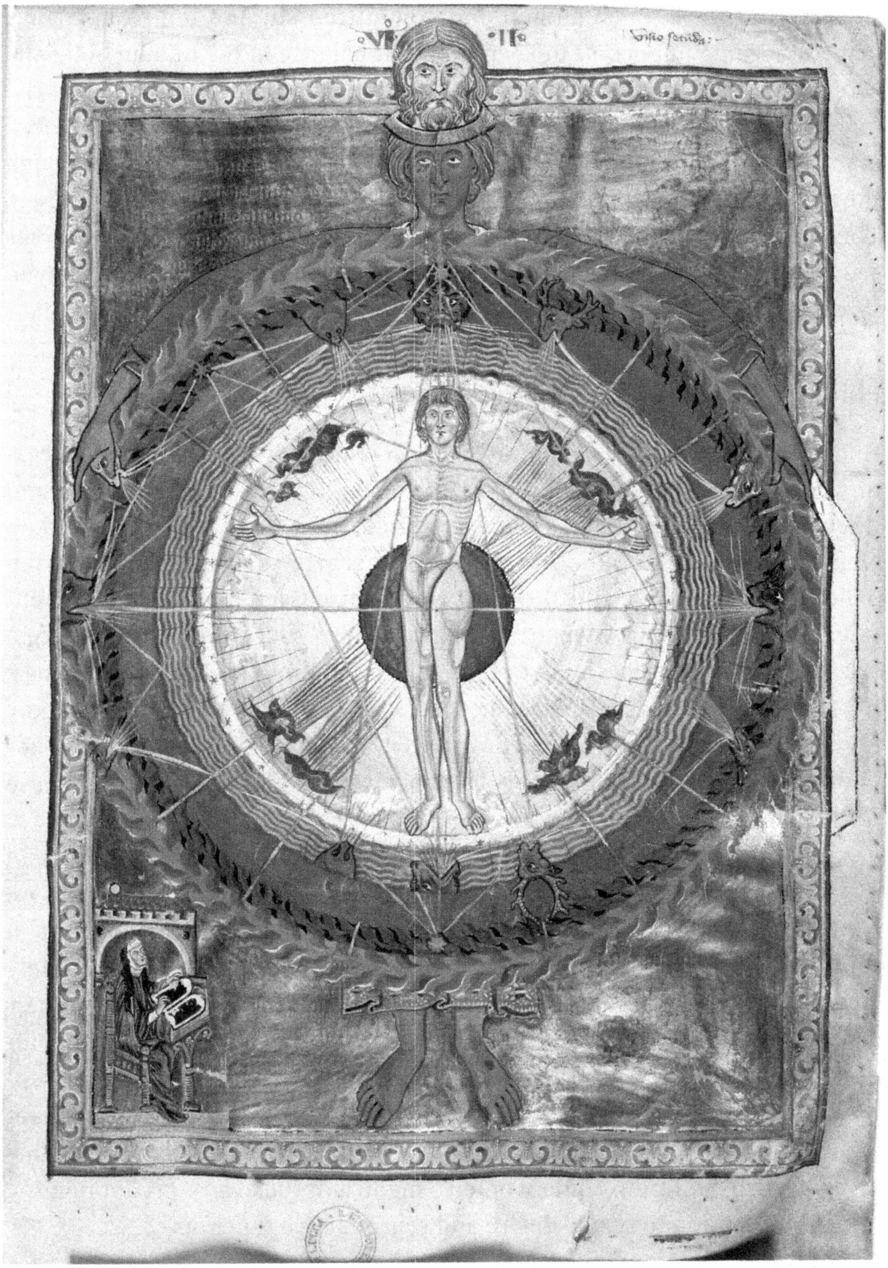

Figure 2. "The Creation with the Universe and the Cosmic Man." In Hildegard of Bingen, *Liber divinorum operum*, thirteenth century. Lucca, Biblioteca Statale di Lucca, MS 1942, fol. 9r. By permission of the Ministry of Culture—Biblioteca Statale di Lucca. Further reproduction, duplication, dissemination, or publication of this image by any means, whether for profit or not, without the authorization of the Biblioteca Statale di Lucca, is prohibited.

For Hildegard, once humankind committed sin and fell from a pure state, it became important to keep the right balance in the human body, the economy of salvation, the Church, and the whole cosmos in her view of the microcosm and macrocosm.[53] Once they become degenerate and therefore start to move, they kept moving. Just as a woman's body cleans itself through the movement of the blood in her period, so also the firmament cleans itself. This motion is especially highlighted as a "flow" when Hildegard analyzes the woman's body, which goes through menstruation, childbirth, and even salvation.

Hildegard's Counter: Positive Porosity

Hildegard of Bingen advocates how and why this process of womanly purgation can become beneficial not only to women but to all of humankind and the whole world. As we have all degenerated, none of us are better off than women, according to Hildegard, a view that sharply distinguishes her from male theologians or medical theorists who discussed and explained menstrual pollution. While menstrual anxiety is also based on women's porosity, allowing menstrual fluids to flow out to pollute men and other beings, Hildegard sees menstruation as the possibility of purgation and purification. A woman's menstruation is the flow out of a woman's body that cleans her body of food waste. Men do not have this flow, as their bodies burn up these residues with their strong heat.

What traits characterize a woman as a woman in the medieval Christian world? Hildegard of Bingen, like many of her contemporaries, focuses on women's reproductive role, understanding female identity largely through reproductive body parts. Medieval physicians and intellectuals routinely emphasized women's reproductive organs, particularly the womb, and their distinctive physiological makeup, characterized by weakness, fragility, coldness, and dampness. These discussions typically concluded that women represented inferior versions of men in virtually every respect. From both theological and social perspectives, a woman's purpose was understood primarily as bearing children, while women's medical issues were predominantly viewed in relation to sexual desire and reproductive function.

In these fundamental assumptions, Hildegard shares much with other writers of her time. Where she diverges—and this marks her revolutionary contribution—is in her interpretation of these physical characteristics.

53 Kalas, "Hildegard's *Causae et curae*," 2.

From contemporaneous narratives of women's weak and leaky bodies, Hildegard uncovers what might be called positive porosity. She transforms perceived weakness into strength, reinterpreting female physical openness as a divinely ordained capacity for healing and salvation. This reframing would profoundly influence her understanding of women's bodies and their spiritual significance throughout her work.

This examination of female porosity reveals how Hildegard integrates the physical realities of women's bodies with theological representations of divine receptivity. For Hildegard, the body's openness is not a weakness. Rather, it is a foundational principle that enables spiritual transformation and salvation. In this way, medical understanding and theological vision become mutually reinforcing aspects of her perspective.

Chapter 2

THE UNSEALER OF SIN

WHAT IS COMMONLY represented by the woman's body? One of the gender differences attributed to the medieval body is its openness and closedness. The body seems to be more complete, whole, and integrated if it is closed. This closedness is also related to unchangeability. If your body is complete, then because of this completeness, you do not need to change or should not be changed. In the Christian tradition, the first woman's body was so open that she invited sin and its aftermath, including reproduction and death.

As we will see in the rest of this book, women were considered more attuned to receiving influences from outside their bodies and undergoing changes in their bodies as a result of these influences. On one hand, this can mean that the woman's body is weaker, less rigid, and less contained. But on the other hand, the permeability of a woman's body can also enable it to adapt to the environment, acquire what it needs, and dispose of what it has too much of. A woman's adaptability could serve as a woman's power to survive. Furthermore, this flexibility can represent the woman's ability to reproduce. Lastly, it can signify a woman's cooperation in saving the souls of others, because human beings can change their minds and redirect them towards God.

Flexible Eve, Rigid Adam

In medieval texts, Eve often represents fallen human nature and the body in general; however, Hildegard of Bingen sees the potential for human salvation in her, too. Granting that Eve was the first sinner against God's commandment, Hildegard emphasizes instead that Eve made it possible for human beings not only to be doomed to perish, but also to be saved through Jesus.

The differences between Adam and Eve that gave Eve this role began with their creation. Hildegard describes Adam's creation as follows:

> When God created man, it was mud stuck together with water, from which the human being was formed. God sent into that form a fiery and airy breath of life. Man was formed from mud and water. The mud was made flesh from the fire of the breath of life and, from the air of that life-breath, the water

> which stuck the mud together became blood. When God created Adam, the splendor of divinity shone about the lump of mud from which he was created. That mud, when the form had been brought forth, appeared with the outlines of limbs on the outside, and empty on the inside.[1]

Here, Hildegard describes how God created Adam with the four elements that compose the universe: not only with mud (earth), but also with water, fire, and air (spirit or breath). At the same time, the four elements are gendered. Earth and fire are more masculine, while air and water are more feminine for Hildegard.[2] Although Adam is created with the four elements, earth and fire are more emphasized and are used to explain Adam's strength and greater sexual desire, which aligns with the traditional view that men have hot and dry natures. Eve is described as more airy and watery, also aligning with the medieval notion that women are cold and wet.

When Adam was created, just as when Eve was later created, the human body did not have any inherent flaws. Adam's bodily members and organs functioned properly. However, Hildegard describes how human beings were changed both physically and mentally after the first transgression:

> God created the human being, and all animals were subject to serving him; but when man transgressed God's order, he was changed in mind and body. The purity of his blood changed to another type, so that instead of purity, it throws off the foam of semen. If the human had stayed in paradise, he would have continued in his unchangeable and perfect state. But these all changed after the transgression into another, bitter type.[3]

---

1 Hildegard of Bingen, *Causes and Cures*, trans. Throop, 35. "Nam cum deus hominem crearet, limus per aquam conglutinatus est, ex quo homo formatus est, misitque deus in formam illam 'spiraculum uite' igneum et aereum. Et quia forma hominis ex limo et aqua fuit, ex igne eiusdem spiraculi uite limus caro factus est, et ex aere eius aqua, per quam limus conglutinatus est, sanguis effecta est. Cum enim deus Adam crearet, splendor diuinitatis massam limi, de qua creatus est, circumfulsit, et ita limus ille illata forma in liniamentis membrorum exterius apparuit et interius uacua." Hildegard of Bingen, *Beate Hildegardis Cause et cure*, ed. Moulinier and Berndt, bk. 2, §76, p. 71.

2 Sur, *Feminine Images of God*, 71.

3 Hildegard of Bingen, *Causes and Cures*, trans. Throop, 28. "Deus ita creauit hominem, quod omnia animalia ad seruitutem eius subiecta sunt; sed cum homo preceptum dei transgressus est, mutatus est etiam tam corpore quam mente. Nam puritas sanguinis eius in alium modum uersa est, ita quod pro puritate spumam seminis eicit. Si enim homo in paradyse mansisset, in inmutabili et perfecto statu perstitisset. Sed hec omnia post transgressionem in alium et amarum modum uersa sunt." Hildegard of Bingen, *Beate Hildegardis Cause et cure*, ed. Moulinier and Berndt, bk. 2, §56, p. 59.

According to Hildegard, it was after the fall that human beings became vulnerable to sickness and phlegm: "Certain people suffer various illnesses from phlegm, which abounds in them. If the human being had remained in paradise, they would not have phlegm, whence many illnesses proceed, in their body. Their flesh would be unimpaired and without darkness (*livore*)."[4] Once fallen, human bodies lost their integrity and became ulcerated and perforated, which invited illness into human bodies.[5]

While the fall changed the physical and psychological conditions of both Eve and Adam, it is interesting that Hildegard lays special emphasis on the adverse changes to Adam's seed in *Cause et cure*: "Partaking of evil, the blood of the sons of Adam transformed into poisonous semen, from which the sons of men are procreated."[6] It seems that in Hildegard's *Cause et cure*, it was mostly Adam whose body changed after the sin and fall. Just before explaining Eve's evil deeds, Hildegard states that Eve's body was not changed as much because she was soft, having been born out of Adam's flesh, while Adam was created with earthly elements. Because Eve was created second and thus indirectly, her body was less affected by the fall:

> After his first sleep, Adam's prophecy was true, since he had not yet sinned; later it was mixed with falsehood. And Adam, created from earth and roused by the elements, was changed, but Eve, created from Adam's rib, was not changed.[7]

---

4 Modified from Hildegard of Bingen, *Causes and Cures*, trans. Throop, 30. "Quod autem quidam homines diuersas infirmitates patiuntur, hoc de flecmate est, quod in ipsis habundat. Si enim homo in paradyso permansisset, flecmata in corpore suo non haberet, unde multa mala procedunt, sed caro eius integra esset et absque liuore." Hildegard of Bingen, *Beate Hildegardis Cause et cure*, ed. Moulinier and Berndt, bk. 2, §64, pp. 63–64.

5 Hildegard of Bingen, *Causes and Cures*, trans. Throop, 31 "Et ideo caro eorum, ulcerata et perforata est. Quae ulcera et foramina quondam tempestatem et humectatem fumi in hominibus faciunt, de quo flecmata oriuntur et coagulantur, que diuersas infirmitates corporibus hominum inferunt." Hildegard of Bingen, *Beate Hildegardis Cause et cure*, ed. Moulinier and Berndt, bk. 2, §64, p. 64.

6 Hildegard of Bingen, *Causes and Cures*, trans. Throop, 31. "Nam de gustu mali uersus est sanguis filiorum Ade in uenenum seminis, de quo filii hominum procreantur." Hildegard of Bingen, *Beate Hildegardis Cause et cure*, ed. Moulinier and Berndt, bk. 2, §64, p. 64.

7 Hildegard of Bingen, *Causes and Cures*, trans. Throop, 38. "Post primum namque sompnum Ade prophetia eius uera fuit, quoniam nondum peccauerat, sed postea cum mendacio permixta est. Et Adam de terra creatus et cum elementis suscitatus mutabatur, Eua uero de costa Ade mutata non est." Hildegard of Bingen, *Beate Hildegardis Cause et cure*, ed. Moulinier and Berndt, bk. 2, §88, p. 77.

After suggesting that Eve's bodily state was less changed than Adam's, Hildegard seems to turn to a discussion of Eve's sin in the next section, but she does not say much about Eve's sin, only mentioning Eve's softness and her role as the mother of the entire human species:

> Adam was virile from the vital force of the earth and very strong from the elements. Eve, from his marrow, was soft[8] and had an airy, keen mind and a pleasant life, since the weight of the earth did not oppress her. Just as she came forth from a man, so all humankind proceeded from her.[9]

After this passage, Hildegard goes on to explain the complementary relationship between waking and sleeping, without mentioning Eve's evil deeds at all. According to the passage above, the primary feature distinguishing Eve from Adam is her softness, which Hildegard does not particularly blame her for. Rather, Eve's soft and delicate nature comes from Adam's marrow. Moreover, this softness and mild nature enabled Eve and her female descendants to have children.[10]

In the next section, on the other hand, about Adam's exile, Hildegard returns to the topic of Adam's sin and his changed state afterwards. Overall, it seems that Hildegard mentions Adam much more often than Eve when she explains the aftereffects of human beings' transgression against God's command. Before the transgression, the human body was able to maintain the right humoral balance. But after the transgression (Hildegard refers to Adam in particular here), people are changed: "Heat, humidity, blood, and flesh are changed into contrary phlegm in people after the transgression of Adam."[11]

---

8 According to Paul Kaiser's 1903 Latin version, which has subheadings for each section, this part is introduced as "De Evae malitia," "Regarding Eve's malice," which was translated by Throop as "Eve's Disposition." However, the passage is mainly about the soft body of Eve; therefore, it is possible that "malitia" is a misspelling of "mollitia," which is "softness." Hildegard of Bingen, *Hildegardis Causae et curae*, ed. Kaiser, 46; Hildegard of Bingen, *Causes and Cures*, trans. Throop, 38.

9 Hildegard of Bingen, *Causes and Cures*, trans. Throop, 38–39. "Et idem Adam de uiriditate terre uirilis et de elementis fortissimus erat, Eua autem de medullis suis mollis fuit et aeream mentem ac acutam artem et deliciosam uitam habuit, quoniam pondus terre eam non pressit. Sed ut ipsa de uiro est educta, sic omne genus humanum ex ipsa processit." Hildegard of Bingen, *Beate Hildegardis Cause et cure*, ed. Moulinier and Berndt, bk. 2, §89, p. 77.

10 Sur, *Feminine Images of God*, 85.

11 Hildegard of Bingen, *Causes and Cures*, trans. Throop, 42. "Calor enim ac humiditas <et> sanguis et caro propter transgressionem Ade in contraria flegmata in homine mutata sunt." Hildegard of Bingen, *Beate Hildegardis Cause et cure*, ed. Moulinier and Berndt, bk. 2, §97, p. 84.

It was Adam's transgression which brought darkness and shadows into the world.[12] In Hildegard's descriptions, Adam seems more responsible not only for his changed state but also for the whole world's mutation.

Even when Hildegard explains why Eve, not Adam, was the first sinner, she does not blame Eve for being a weak woman. It was God who created Eve in this way, and it was Adam who gave her softness and malleability from his own body:

> If Adam had transgressed before Eve, the transgression would have been so strong and incorrigible that man would have fallen in such greatly hardened incorrigibility that he would neither wish, nor be able, to be saved. Because Eve transgressed first, it was able to be more easily nullified, since she was weaker than a male. The flesh and skin of Adam was harder and stronger than that of men now, because Adam was formed from earth, and Eve from him. After they produced children, flesh became always weaker and weaker, and thus it will be until the last day.[13]

According to Hildegard, human beings would not have had any chance for salvation if Adam had sinned first, because his rigidity would have made the transgression "incorrigible." This notion implies a negative side to his strength. In this logic, Eve's softness makes it rather fortunate for humankind that she sinned.[14] Of course, Hildegard derives this contrast of hard-

12 "After Adam sinned, night began to be present, and all elements were overshadowed by great darkness; in this darkness, Adam was led into exile." Hildegard of Bingen, *Causes and Cures*, trans. Throop, 39. "Sed postquam Adam peccauit, nox adesse cepit, et omnia elementa magnis tenebris obtenebrata sunt, in quibus Adam in exilium istud deductus est." Hildegard of Bingen, *Beate Hildegardis Cause et cure*, ed. Moulinier and Berndt, bk. 2, §90, p. 78.

13 Hildegard of Bingen, *Causes and Cures*, trans. Throop, 39. "Sed et si Adam transgressus fuisset prius quam Eua, tunc transgressio illa tam fortis et tam incorrigibilis fuisset, quod homo etiam in tam magna obduratione incorrigibilitatis cecidisset, quod nec saluari uellet nec posset. Vnde quod Eua prior transgrediebatur, facilius deleri potuit, quia etiam fragilior masculo fuit. Caro et cutis Ade et Eue fortior et durior fuit quam hominum nunc sit, quia Adam de terra formatus fuit et Eue de ipso. Sed postquam filios genuerunt, caro illorum semper et semper fragilior et fragilior facta est, et ita usque in nouissimum diem erit." Hildegard of Bingen, *Beate Hildegardis Cause et cure*, ed. Moulinier and Berndt, bk. 2, §91, p. 79. It should be noted that the Berndt and Moulinier Latin edition reads "Caro et cutis Ade et Eue" while Throop's translation only renders "[t]he flesh and skin of Adam," omitting Eve. This discrepancy arises because Throop bases her translation on Kaiser's edition, as she indicates in her introduction, where the text appears as "Caro et cutis Adae" without reference to Eve. See Hildegard of Bingen, *Hildegardis Causae et curae*, ed. Kaiser, 47.

14 Barbara Newman's suggestion that Jesus's humanity originated from Eve's

ness and malleability from physiological explanations: Adam was made of earth, and Eve was made of Adam's soft flesh. Eve's softness is thus not in itself a bad or particularly female feature, considering that this softness came from Adam.

Also, women were provided with a tremendous opportunity to take revenge on evil through their own bodies when the Virgin Mary bore the Saviour and sent him out into the world: "the ancient serpent was greatly terrified and astounded, because he had been wholly deceived by a woman—the Virgin."[15] Whereas the first woman's malleable body allowed sin to enter humankind, the Virgin's porous body brought salvation to human beings by receiving the Holy Spirit, becoming pregnant, and giving birth to the Saviour. In this history of the Fall and Salvation, the woman's body is highlighted. It is the woman's body that receives sin and has the opportunity to nullify sin. The woman's body is like a garment that the Virgin Mary receives from the Saviour as a theophany, since her body has the ability to store him.[16]

Hildegard's positive depiction of female bodies in *Cause et cure* is unsurprising in light of her positive presentation of Eve in the first book of *Scivias*. In Vision Two of Book One, Hildegard presents her account of the Fall.[17] One interesting thing about Hildegard's depiction of the Fall is the way that the original sin changed the entire bodily system of human beings. The beautiful bodies of human beings lost their peaceful state after

---

weakness in fact reinforces Ecclesia by compounding strength and weakness as well as divinity and humanity. Newman, *Sister of Wisdom*, 182.

15 This is Hildegard's exegesis of Revelation 12:13–14. Hildegard of Bingen, *Book of Divine Works*, trans. Campbell, 286. "Quoniam [antiquus serpens] per mulierem, uidelicet uirginem, totus deceptus est." Hildegard of Bingen, *Liber divinorum operum*, ed. Derolez and Dronke, pt. 2, bk. 1, chap. 16, p. 284.

16 Newman, *Sister of Wisdom*, 90–93.

17 Hildegard of Bingen, *Scivias*, trans. Hart and Bishop, 73. "DEINDE VIDI uelut maximam multitudinem uiuentium lampadarum multam claritatem habentium, quae igneum fulgorem accipientes ita serenissimum splendorem adeptae sunt. Et ecce lacus multae latitudinis et profunditatis apparuit, os uelut os putei habens et igneum fumum cum multo foetore emittens, de quo etiam taeterrima nebula se extendens quasi uenam uisum deceptibilem habentem tetigit, et in quadam clara regione candidam nubem quae de quadam pulchra forma hominis plurimas plurimasque stellas in se continens exierat per eam afflauit ac illam eandemque formam hominis de eadem regione ita eiecit. Quo facto lucidissimus splendor eandem regionem circumdedit, et ita omnia elementa mundi, quae prius in magna quiete constiterant, in maximam inquietudinem uersa horribiles terrores ostenderunt." Hildegard of Bingen, *Scivias*, ed. Führkötter and Carelvaris, pt. 1, bk. 2, chap. 73, p. 13.

the Fall. Before Adam and Eve picked the forbidden fruit, their bodies were perfect. When their bodies were perfect, they did not need to procreate. But because they were expelled from Paradise and eternal life, they began to need to have intercourse and have children. In the exegesis that follows this description, Hildegard explains it in terms of God's creation as well as the fall of Adam and Eve. Of course, Adam and Eve disobeyed God and thus committed the original sin, but Hildegard does not necessarily blame Eve for introducing sin to humanity, although she does not deny that it happened because of Eve's weakness. She concedes that Eve's weakness originated from God's deliberate creation, which begot women's weakness in general. Women are made softer so that they can receive semen from men. Women's weakness and softness are thus by God's design and absolutely necessary for generation.[18]

Because women were created in this way, their weakness, understood as necessary softness, was not something blameworthy. This could be another reason why Adam did not blame Eve, according to Hildegard, since Eve was born weak. Hildegard interprets the story of Adam and Eve as a model for why husbands and wives have to love each other, rather than blame Eve for the origin of sin. Even though Eve introduced Adam and all of his offspring to death and sin, her horrible mistake does not separate her from her husband. What else could make a husband leave his wife, if not this, Hildegard seems to ask. Hildegard thus turns the narrative of Eve's sin into one about marriage—a story of the love and bond between men and women.

> Because he [the Devil] knew that the susceptibility of the woman would be more easily conquered than the strength of the man; and he saw that Adam burned so vehemently in his holy love for Eve that if he, the Devil, conquered Eve, Adam would do whatever she said to him . . . [the Devil acted] by first misleading Eve, so that she might flatter and caress Adam and thus win his assent, since she more than any other creature could lead Adam to

18 Hildegard of Bingen, *Scivias*, trans. Hart and Bishop, 77. "Sed sicut non paruo puero sed perfecto uiro, scilicet Adae, perfecta mulier data est, ita etiam modo, cum uir in perfecta aetate sua fertilis est, perfecta ei mulier coniungenda est, uelut cum arbor flores incipit emittere debita cultura ei adhibenda est. Nam de costa insito calore et suco Adae Eua formata est, ac ideo nunc de fortitudine uiri et de calore eius semen mulier concipit prolem in mundum producere. Vir enim seminator existit, mulier autem susceptrix seminis est. Vnde et mulier sub potestate uiri manet, quoniam ut duritia lapidis ad teneritudinem terrae est, ita etiam et fortitudo uiri ad mollitiem mulieris est." Hildegard of Bingen, *Scivias*, ed. Führkötter and Carelvaris, pt. 1, bk. 2, chap. 11, p. 77.

> disobedience, having been made from his rib. Thus woman very quickly overthrows man, if he does not hate her and easily accepts her words.[19]

Hildegard here continues to highlight the love of Eve and Adam. Hildegard even suggests that the first human being's first transgression was due not only to Eve's weak nature, but also to Adam's strong love for Eve. This interpretation differs from that of some theologians, who locate the reason that Eve was deceived in her own weakness. For example, Peter Lombard, a theologian and Hildegard's contemporary, argues that Eve was deceived first due to her "less vigorous" rationality,[20] and that Eve's sin was more serious than Adam's due to her pride.[21]

According to Hildegard, Adam was deceived by the Devil because he loved Eve so much that he had to listen to her. Hildegard did not see his love as something for which Eve should be blamed. Rather, it was only natural that Adam loved Eve so much, because she was born from his own body. The Devil deserves the blame, then, because the Devil abused Eve's susceptibility and Adam's love.

> For Adam could have blamed his wife because by her advice she brought him death, but nonetheless he did not dismiss her as long as he lived in this world, because he knew she had been given to him by divine power. Therefore, because of perfect love, let a man not leave his wife except for the reason the faithful Church allows.[22]

---

19 Hildegard of Bingen, *Scivias*, trans. Hart and Bishop, 77. "Quia sciebat mulieris mollitiem facilius uincendam quam uiri fortitudinem, uidens etiam quod Adam in caritate Euae tam fortiter ardebat ut si ipse diabolus Euam uicisset, quidquid illa Adae diceret, Adam idem perficeret. Vnde et diabolus illam eandemque formam hominis de eadem regione ita eiecit: quoniam idem antiquus seductor Euam atque Adam de sede beatitudinis sua deceptione expellens eos in tenebras subuersionis misit. Quomodo? Videlicet Euam primum seduxit, ut ipsa Adae blandiretur, quatenus ei assensum praeberet, quia ipsa citius Adam quam alia creatura ad inoboedientiam perducere potuit, quoniam de costa illius facta fuerat. Quapropter mulier uirum citius deicit, cum ille eam non abhorrens uerba eius facile assumit." Hildegard of Bingen, *Scivias*, ed. Führkötter and Carelvaris, pt. 1, bk. 2, chap. 10, p. 19.

20 Peter Lombard, *The Sentences: Book 2 on Creation*, trans. Silano, dist. 21, chap. 1, p. 92.

21 Peter Lombard, *The Sentences: Book 2 on Creation*, trans. Silano, dist. 22, chap. 3, p. 100. Here, Lombard argues against Augustine, who said Eve's pride and Adam's pride were equal and therefore their sins were equal.

22 Hildegard of Bingen, *Scivias*, trans. Hart and Bishop, 78. "Adam enim uxorem suam culpare posset quod ei consilio suo mortem intulit, sed tamen eam non dimisit quamdiu in hoc saeculo uixit, quoniam illam sibi per diuinam potentiam datam esse cognouit. Vnde propter perfectam caritatem non relinquat homo

What is interesting here is that Hildegard emphasizes the unbreakable bond of marriage, even in the story of the Fall. Although Eve's earlier transgression could be, and often was, used to support the idea that women should be subjected to men, Hildegard does not see it that way. Instead, Hildegard argues that Eve's behaviour did not make Adam blame or abandon her. For Hildegard, then, it was more important for Adam that Eve was given to him by God. The fact that Adam did not divorce Eve supports Hildegard's logic that husbands and wives should not leave their partners.

In Hildegard's interpretation of the creation story, the bond between men and women precedes women's subjection. Both her vision and Genesis explain that husbands and wives should love each other. But Hildegard also uses the story of Adam and Eve to explain why married people should not cheat on their partners—namely, because wives and husbands were born from the same body, just as Eve was created from Adam's body. Adam's affection towards Eve sometimes appears in medieval theology as a justification for why the serpent approached Eve first and why Adam had to listen to Eve. But Hildegard is unique in drawing from the story a moral lesson about why husbands and wives must have a strong bond.[23]

Eve, Women, and Water

For Hildegard, the image of living water is central, especially since she uses gardens and plants literally and figuratively. For her, water is to be supplied and flow through a garden to grow plants. Moisture in the form of rain, dew, and fountains leads to *viriditas*, an important concept in Hildegard's theology and medicine. In her letter to an abbot who asked for her advice regarding his office, Hildegard gives him advice in the voice of God. Moisture is

---

uxorem suam nisi propter rationabilem causam illam quam sibi fidelis ecclesia proponit." Hildegard of Bingen, *Scivias*, ed. Führkötter and Carelvaris, pt. 1, bk. 2, chap. 11, p. 20.

23 It seems that Adam and Eve's strong bond was emphasized more after the Reformation. Kathleen M. Crowther examines German plays and poems in the Protestant Reformation to show that Adam and Eve's partnership began to be emphasized as a new ideal type of family, partly objecting to the Catholic ideal life of celibacy. See Crowther, *Adam and Eve in the Protestant Reformation*. In the *Glossa ordinaria*, on the other hand, it seems Eve's subordinate status was emphasized rather than Adam and Eve's mutual love. However, Hildegard does not deny that women were subjected to men due to Eve's first transgression.

opposed to bitterness, while wisdom is opposed to grossness and viridity is opposed to labour.[24]

> But you, O friend of the grace of God, you have a garden of people, in which as the representative of Christ you seek to plant many wholesome desires and good works. And through the power of His gifts, the grace of God pours out His dynamic good will upon those desires and those works, and causes the garden to grow green through the dew and the rain of the fountain of living water.[25]

For Hildegard, virtues are the plants of God, and the plants need to be watered. Women can fulfil this duty, in part because their bodies are wetter, according to medieval physiology. But their knowledge can also contribute to their power, as Sweet notes when discussing the importance of the garden and the gardener in Hildegard's medicine and theology.[26] The gardener is Hildegard, who collected healing knowledge to cure people with herbs, as many women did.

On the other hand, the Virgin Mary is often referred to as an ever-flowing fountain and a sealed garden, which is not far from the watering image. In his exegesis of the Song of Songs, Honorius of Autun, a theologian and Hildegard's contemporary, explains that the Virgin Mary was the fountain who received and emitted Jesus through her body: "As the Jordan flowed from the mountains, he who consecrated the font of baptism for the world flowed from her womb."[27] The image of the fountain is strongly tied to Hildegard's emphasis on baptism. As Newman says, "[t]he womb" of the Church is the baptismal font, fertilized and sanctified by the Spirit—an act dramatically symbolized at the consecration of the font, when the paschal candle is plunged into the water.[28]

The image of the fountain is not just limited to the Virgin Mary, however, and Newman also points out the importance of fountains in Hildegard's understanding of women.[29] For example, in her response to Archbishop Hillinus of Trier, who was seeking her comforting words, Hildegard refers

24 "Hildegard to Adam, the Abbot," in Hildegard of Bingen, *Letters*, trans. Baird and Ehrman, no. 85r/b, 1:195.

25 "Hildegard to Adam, the Abbot," in Hildegard of Bingen, *Letters*, trans. Baird and Ehrman, no. 85r/b, 1:195.

26 Sweet, *Rooted in the Earth*.

27 Honorius, *The Seal of Blessed Mary*, trans. Carr, 51.

28 Newman, *Sister of Wisdom*, 189.

29 Newman, *Sister of Wisdom*, 98.

to women as fountains when encouraging him to perform his office in this "squalid, womanish time (*squalidum tempus muliebris*)." Even when man has more strength, "woman is a fountain of wisdom and a fountain of plenty of joy, which parts man brings to perfection."[30] Both Hildegard and Hillinus acknowledge Hildegard as being a woman and weak. And at the same time, both know that her weakness becomes a strong point.[31] While women are weak, this weakness makes it possible for women to be filled with sacred knowledge and joy, drawing them towards perfection. Even the first woman, Eve, was compared to a fountain in relation to Adam.[32]

Virginity: Sealed vs. Porous

The weak body is also associated with porosity. Its weakness means that it is breakable and something that can be invaded. In medieval Christianity and medicine, this porosity caused by weakness was treated negatively. It was the sign of imperfection, always receiving and sending out something. This weak, porous image also applies to the Hildegardian physiology that women are more susceptible to health issues related to sexual activities and reproductive processes.[33] But even when the woman's body was generally considered weak and porous, there were different levels of porosity. And it was often supported by the physical state of virginity. Especially when the woman's sexual experience was described as "rupture," the virginal body was the one which was relatively less porous. And the virginal body of Mary before and after giving birth to Jesus was more tightly sealed.

---

30 Modified from "Hildegard to Hillinus, Archbishop of Trier," in Hildegard of Bingen, *Letters*, trans. Baird and Ehrman, no. 26r, 1:88. "Mulier autem est fons sapientiae et fons pleni gaudii, quas partes vir ad perfectum ducit." Hildegard of Bingen, *S. Hildegardis Abbatissae Opera omnia*, ed. Migne, chap. 13, p. 167B.

31 "It has pleased the wisdom of God, which chooses 'the weak things of the world that he may confound the strong' [I Cor 1.27]." "Hillinus, Archbishop of Trier, to Hildegard," in Hildegard of Bingen, *Letters*, trans. Baird and Ehrman, no. 26, 1:87.

32 Hildegard of Bingen, *Causes and Cures*, trans. Throop, 111. "Magna autem dilectio, que in Adam erat, cum Eua de ipso exiuit, et dulcedo soporis illius, qua tunc dormiuit, in transgressione eius in contrarium modum dulcedinis uersa est. Et ideo, quia uir hanc magnam dulcedinem in se sentit et habet, ut 'ceruus ad fontem,' sic ipse uelociter ad feminam currit et femina ad ipsum in similitudine horrei aree, que multis ictibus percutitur et ad calorem perducitur, cum grana in ea excutiuntur." Hildegard of Bingen, *Beate Hildegardis Cause et cure*, ed. Moulinier and Berndt, bk. 2, §283, p. 176.

33 Cadden, "It Takes All Kinds," 171.

Sarah Salih examines the complexity of meanings and practices attached to the virginal body in the Middle Ages. In her *Versions of Virginity in Late Medieval England*, Salih introduces different levels of virginity. She argues that virginity can be achieved through an invincible precondition, communal life, and re-imagined physical states.[34] For example, the Virgin Mary's undoubted integrity needs to be approached differently than Hildegard and her nuns' monastic virginity. While the Virgin Mary's keeping of her virginity before, during, and after giving birth to Christ is impossible to achieve for other women, her existence and presence in the Christian tradition opened the gates for Christian women to be centred in Christian traditions and discourses regarding the body.

Medieval Christianity emphasizes the Virgin Mary's fertile and pure body as a sealed fountain. Mary's virginal body is often referred to as closed and sealed against evil, sexual activity, and any form of sin. For example, Origen relates the closed body of the Virgin Mary to the closed gate in Ezekiel[35] in order to support her virginity from the more profound authority of Hebrew Scripture.[36] But even the most sealed woman, the Virgin Mary, has a certain level of porosity. While she is known to have had no physical contact with men, she certainly received the Holy Spirit in her body. In Marian devotion, her body is understood as sealed against the male seed but touched by the Holy Spirit. Although the body of the Saviour's mother should be sealed, it should also be open to receive the Holy Spirit and store it until the child's delivery. Honorius of Autun, Hildegard's contemporary theologian, praises the sealed nature of Mary's body in his exegesis of the Song of Songs,[37] a biblical book that, despite its complicated symbolism and meanings, provides an important opportunity for women to be the centre of its allegorical interpretations.[38] However, at the same time, Honorius focuses on Mary being a sealed "fountain," suggesting that things flow in and out of her despite the

---

34 Salih, *Versions of Virginity*, 1–2.

35 "Then said the LORD unto me; This gate shall be shut, it shall not be opened, and no man shall enter in by it; because the LORD, the God of Israel, hath entered in by it, therefore it shall be shut." Ezekiel 44:2–3.

36 Rubin, *Mother of God*, 55.

37 Honorius, *The Seal of Blessed Mary*, trans. Carr, 51–52.

38 McAvoy has focused on the symbolism of the garden in explaining the importance of women and their wombs as represented in the Song of Songs. See "Chapter One: Out of Eden: The Framing of Eve" in McAvoy, *The Enclosed Garden*.

seal. Similarly, the Virgin Mary was referred to as the window of heaven, which can receive the "sun of justice shone into the house of the world."[39]

Miri Rubin also emphasizes the Virgin Mary's Annunciation scene and points out the characteristics of Annunciation scenes.[40] The Annunciation usually happens in a closed room where the Archangel Gabriel delivers the news. This enclosed space, however, has windows through which a dove, signifying the Holy Spirit, sometimes enters. While the windows might have various shapes and positions, some important illustrations show that the Virgin Mary receives the Holy Spirit through the window. These depictions represent the various levels of permeability that characterized even the most closed woman. The woman's body cannot be completely sealed off even when she keeps her virginity. When women keep their bodies virginal, they are closed to men while they are still open to the Holy Spirit.

Woman as Vessel

Hildegard represents the woman's body as a vessel, permeable to different fluids and able to contain a foetus as well as semen; her *Scivias* also represents the womb as a vessel, but one permeable to spiritual substances and able to contain souls. Admittedly, the idea of the physical vessel is to some extent applicable to males as well. For example, Hildegard depicts human bodies in general as containers in Vision Four of Book One of *Scivias*, where she describes the souls and bodies of human beings:

> And behold! I saw on the earth people carrying milk in earthen vessels and making cheeses from it; and one part was thick, and from it strong cheeses were made; and one part was thin, and from it weak cheeses were curdled; and one part was mixed with corruption, and from it bitter cheeses were formed.[41]

Here Hildegard describes the human figures in her vision as holding vessels full of milk, which she goes on to explain represents the "human seed." Indeed, in her exegesis of this vision, Hildegard draws an analogy between human conception and the process of milk being turned into different cheeses.

---

39 Honorius, *The Seal of Blessed Mary*, trans. Carr, 209.

40 Rubin, *Mother of God*, 342–45.

41 Hildegard of Bingen, *Scivias*, trans. Hart and Bishop, 109. "Et ecce uidi in terra homines in uasis suis lac portantes et inde caseos facientes, cuius quaedam pars spissa fuit, unde fortes casei facti sunt, pars quaedam tenuis, de qua debiles casei coagulate sunt, et pars quaedam tabe permixta, de qua amari casei effecti sunt." Hildegard of Bingen, *Scivias*, ed. Führkötter and Carelvaris, pt. 1, bk. 4, p. 61.

> *You see also on the earth people carrying milk in earthen vessels and making cheese from it*; these are the people in the world, both men and women, who have in their bodies human seed, from which the various races of people are procreated. *One part is thick, and from it strong cheeses are made*; for that strong semen, which is usefully and well matured and tempered, produces energetic people, to whom brilliant spiritual and bodily gifts are given by their great and noble ancestors, making them flourish in prudence, discretion and usefulness in their works before God and Man, and the Devil finds no place in them. *And one part is thin, and from it weak cheeses are curdled*; for this semen, imperfectly matured and tempered in a weak season, produces weak people, who are for the most part foolish, languid and useless in their works in the sight of God and the world, not actively seeking God. But also *one part is mixed with corruption, and from it bitter cheeses are formed*; for that semen is basely emitted in weakness and confusion and mixed uselessly, and it produces misshapen people, who often have bitterness, adversity and oppression of heart and are thus unable to raise their minds to higher things.[42]

Hildegard makes it clear through her explanation of this vision that people with their seed are like vessels holding milk: from the nature of each one's milk, different kinds and qualities of people can emerge. The important feature of this vision is that Hildegard represents the human bodies of both sexes as vessel-like containers of essential reproductive materials. Whether man or woman, each person has a body like a vessel containing their differently decocted seed, each with its own nature like different cheeses.

42 Hildegard of Bingen, *Scivias*, trans. Hart and Bishop, 118. "Vides etiam in terra homines in uasis suis lac portantes et inde caseos facientes: qui sunt in mundo homines, tam uiri quam mulieres, in corporibus suis humanum semen habentes, de quo genus diuersorum populorum procreatur; cuius quaedam pars spissa est, unde fortes casei fiunt: quia semen illud in fortitudine sua utiliter et bene coctum et temperatum strenuos homines producit, quibus etiam magna claritas tam spiritalium quam carnalium donorum in magnis patribus et in altis personis tribuitur, ita quod in prosperitate prudentiae, discretionis et utilitatis in operibus suis et coram Deo et coram hominibus perspicue florent, quoniam diabolus in eis locum suum non inuenit. Et pars quaedam tenuis de qua debiles casei coagulantur: quoniam hoc semen in teneritudine sua inutiliter semicoctum et semitemperatum teneros homines educit, ita quod isti multoties stulti, tepidi et inutiles tam apud Deum quam apud saeculum in operibus suis sunt, quia Deum strenue non quaerunt. Sed et pars quaedam tabe permixta est, de qua amari casei efficiuntur, quia semen illud in debilitate permixtionis nequiter eductum et inutiliter commixtum informes homines efficit, ita quod illi saepe amaritudinem, difficultatem et oppressionem cordis habent, unde mentem suam multoties ad superiora leuare non ualent." Hildegard of Bingen, *Scivias*, ed. Führkötter and Carelvaris, pt. 1, bk. 4, chap. 13, pp. 75–76.

However, when Hildegard comes to the female process of childbirth, she emphasizes the womb as a vessel capable of containing more than just fluids or physical substances. The process of the ensoulment of any embryo involves a kind of spiritual transfer because the independent life of the body only begins when the soul enters the embryo. It is clear that Hildegard sees this as a divine process, and the soul when it enters the womb is in a divinely pristine state, as her exegesis indicates:

> *And you see the image of a woman who has a perfect human form in her womb.* This means that after a woman has conceived by human semen, an infant with all its members whole is formed in the secret chamber of her womb. And behold! *By the secret design of the Supernal Creator that form moves with vital motion*; for, by God's secret and hidden command and will, fitly and rightly at the divinely appointed time the infant in the maternal womb receives a spirit, and shows by the movements of its body that it lives, just as the earth opens and brings forth the flowers of its use when the dew falls on it. *So that a fiery globe which has no human lineaments possesses the heart of that form*; that is, the soul, burning with a fire of profound knowledge, which discerns whatever is within the circle of its understanding, and, without the form of human members, since it is not corporeal or transitory like a human body, gives strength to the heart and rules the whole body as its foundation, as the firmament of Heaven contains the lower regions and touches the higher.[43]

In this passage, Hildegard echoes in ecstatic terms her description of ensoulment in *Cause et cure*. The pristine soul, envisioned as a fiery globe as it enters "the secret chamber" of the womb, performs the mystery of its life-giving function, animating the members and touching the brain. In this way, the womb becomes almost a holy of holies, a sacred container. Having a

---

43 Hildegard of Bingen, *Scivias*, trans. Hart and Bishop, 119–20. "Sed quod uides quasi mulierem uelut integram formam hominis in utero suo habentem: hoc est quia postquam femina humanum semen conceperit, in integritate membrorum suorum infans in abdito cubiculo uentris ipsius formatur. Et ecce per secretam dispositionem superni conditoris eadem forma motum uiuidae motionis dat: quoniam cum in secreta et occulta iussione et uoluntate Dei infans in materno utero congruo et recte diuinitus disposito tempore spiritum acceperit, motu corporis sui se uiuere ostendit, uelut terra se aperit et flores fructus sui profert cum ros super eam ceciderit, ita quod uelut ignea sphaera nulla lineamenta humani corporis habens cor eiusdem formae possidet: quia anima in igne profundae scientiae ardens diuersas res circuitu suae comprehensionis discernit nec formam humanorum membrorum habens, quoniam ipsa nec corporea nec caduca quemadmodum corpus hominis est, cor hominis confortat, quod quasi fundamentum corporis existens totum corpus regit, uelut firmamentum caeli inferiora continet et superiora tegit." Hildegard of Bingen, *Scivias*, ed. Führkötter and Carelvaris, pt. 1, bk. 4, chap. 16, pp. 77–78.

womb, women are thus represented as permeable to the divinely pure substance of the soul as well as the normal fluids of blood and semen.

As we have seen, Hildegard also describes the human body in *Cause et cure* as a container of the soul. In *Scivias*, she places this concept in the context of the whole process of creation and embodied human experience:

> The Law is ordained for human salvation, and the prophets show forth the hidden things of God; so also human senses protect a person from harmful things and lay bare the soul's interior. For the soul emanates the senses. How? It vivifies a person's face and glorifies him with sight, hearing, taste, smell, and touch, so that by this touch he becomes watchful in all things. For the senses are the sign of all the powers of the soul, as the body is the vessel of the soul. *How? The senses close all the powers of the soul.* What does this mean? A person is recognized by his face, sees with his eyes, hears with his ears, opens his mouth to speak, feels with his hands, walks with his feet; and so the senses are to a person as precious stones and as a rich treasure sealed in a vase. But as the treasure within is known when the vase is seen, so also the powers of the soul are inferred by the senses.[44]

This vision presents the body as the vessel of the soul. A person engages with the world by using their eyes, mouth, hands, and feet. This is only possible because the soul sits in the body. The soul in turn receives sensory input through the bodily members, enabling consciousness and judgment. Hildegard describes the soul in the body as being like precious stones in a sealed vase (or container). According to Hildegard, when you see a sealed vase, you assume that there are jewels inside, because a vase is supposed to contain and protect a valuable thing. Likewise, if you see a human body, you can expect it to contain the precious treasure of a soul.

---

44 The Latin in the footnote has "Quomodo? Sensus omnes uires animae claudit" which is missing from the English translation. I have added this omitted passage in italics: "Therefore, I placed my translation in italic: "How? The senses close all the powers of the soul." Hildegard of Bingen, *Scivias*, trans. Hart and Bishop, 123. "Lex ad salutem hominis posita est, et prophetae occulta Dei manifestant, sic et sensus hominis quaeque nociua ab homine depellit et interiora animae denudat. Nam anima sensum exspirat. Quomodo? Ipsa hominem uiuente facie uiuificat et uisu, auditu, gustu, odoratu et tactu glorificat, ita quod homo sensu tactus peruigil in omnibus rebus fit. Sensus enim signum omnium uirium animae est, sicut et corpus uas animae est. Quomodo? Sensus omnes uires animae claudit. Quid est hoc? Homo in facie cognoscitur, oculis uidet, auribus audit, os ad loquendum aperit, manibus palpat, pedibus ambulat et ideo sensus est in homine uelut pretiosi lapides et ut pretiosus thesaurus in uase signatus. Sed ut uas uidetur et ut in eo thesaurus scitur, ita etiam in sensu ceterae uires animae intelleguntur." Hildegard of Bingen, *Scivias*, ed. Führkötter and Carelvaris, pt. 1, bk. 4, chap. 24, p. 83.

Hildegard believed that the body became a container for the soul while in the mother's womb. When a woman receives a man's semen and holds it until it comes into contact with the menstrual materials, the womb becomes a container for the foetus. More importantly, the womb's shelter helps the developing foetus become a container for the soul made and implanted by God. In explaining this process, Hildegard emphasizes how the womb always serves as a container for something slightly miraculous, even in ordinary childbirth. This image of the womb as a vessel for something divine is an important motif throughout *Scivias* and Hildegard's theological understanding of human beings, as it represents her sense that the womb always mediates the flow of life by receiving and emitting a soul. Hildegard treats all kinds of flow associated with birth as essentially divine and vital:

> For as Man was born in the flesh when divine power created him in the form of Adam, so the Holy Spirit revives the life of the soul by the pouring out of water; It receives into Itself the spirit of the person, restoring him to life, as he is first brought into life on a wave of blood when he comes out of the vessel of the body. And just as a human form is then lovingly formed and called human, so now the soul of the person is vivified in water before the eyes of God, so that God knows that he is an inheritor of life.[45]

In this passage, Hildegard describes baptism as analogous to birth: the flow of water is analogous to the flow of blood during childbirth as the baby exits the vessel of the womb. Here God's grace and a mother's delivery of her child are drawn together as parts of a single sacred process.

These examples suggest that in *Scivias*, Hildegard depicts the human body, and a woman's body in particular, as an important vessel for the soul. Of course, according to Hildegard, the most perfect example of the body as a vessel is the Virgin Mary, who conceived and bore Jesus in her womb. However, in all cases, this positive description of the human body as a vessel is strongly connected to Hildegard's depiction in *Cause et cure* of the body as the container of the soul. Grounded in her medical knowledge, Hildegard presents a positive, and even sacred, image of the womb as bringing forth

45 Hildegard of Bingen, *Scivias*, trans. Hart and Bishop, 181–82. "Nam sicut homo nascitur ex carne, diuina potestate in forma Adae illum creante, ita Spiritus sanctus recuperat uitam animae per inundationem aquae, cum ipsa spiritum hominis in se accipit eum resuscitans ad uitam, ut prius in unda sanguinis suscitatus est, cum in corporali uasculo manifestatus est. Vt enim forma hominis tunc amabiliter formatur, ita quod homo dicitur, sic spiritus hominis ante oculos Dei nunc in aqua uiuificatur, ita quod eum Deus ad hereditatem uitae nouit." Hildegard of Bingen, *Scivias*, ed. Führkötter and Carelvaris, pt. 2, bk. 3, chap. 30, p. 153.

not only the miraculous souls and bodies of all children, but also human salvation through the body of Jesus.

Hildegard's understanding of Eve and Mary demonstrates that the theological narrative of sin and redemption is deeply rooted in physiological characteristics. Eve's initial flexibility and Mary's receptive virginity both exemplify how bodily vulnerability creates spiritual potentials. Through her close theological and medical examinations, Hildegard challenges the traditional medieval view of female bodies as inherently problematic, instead recasting their porosity as divinely purposeful.

Chapter 3

RELEASING BLOOD AND HUMOURS

SUPPORTED BY RELIGIOUS ideas, medieval medicine tends to describe women's nature as simple and singular, often omitting discussion of their diversity or differences. This tendency especially stands out in comparison to the many medical opinions on men's varied nature and temperaments. Medieval doctors follow the stereotypical belief that women essentially have the same nature as Eve, who was seen as so licentious, lustful, and weak that she was easily deceived by the serpent; differences of humoral composition and temperament from one female to another are often ignored or brushed aside in medieval medical literature. By contrast, Hildegard thoroughly sets out the diversity of women's nature and temperaments, thereby departing from contemporary male medical theorists who did not distinguish among the various proportions of the four temperaments in women.

This approach is important because Hildegard emphasizes gender differences in her temperament theories. For instance, Cadden points out that Hildegard's case is unique in that she did not ignore women in her treatment of the four temperaments or portray women's temperaments as subcategories of men's temperaments. What is more interesting is that her depiction of sexual differences in the four temperaments is closely connected to her view that women and men are different from and complementary to each other, raising important issues of anatomy, physiology, sexuality, reproduction, and behaviour across genders in her religious and scientific writings.[1]

The issue of menstruation is a clear example of Hildegard's positive view of the female reproductive body. Some medieval theologians insisted that menstrual fluids were so harmful that intercourse with a woman during menstruation could result in monstrous, leprous, or deformed children.[2] However, Hildegard's reasoning tends to focus on the common humanity of both sexes, which gives her a more positive view of all bodies and bodily processes. Hildegard does not mention the dangerous pollution of menstruation, as male theologians do. Even when she forbids men to have sexual

1 Cadden, *Meanings of Sex Difference*, 153.

2 Langum, *Medicine and the Seven Deadly Sins*, 183.

relationships with menstruating women, it is not about pollution; instead, she sympathizes with women who are already suffering menstrual discomfort. Although menstruation was the punishment from God when Eve transgressed, Hildegard argues that it still should not prevent women from attending church.

Moreover, Hildegard emphasizes the complementary roles of the two sexes in reproduction. In Hildegard's cosmological understanding, Adam's semen became poisonous after he sinned against God. By contrast, women do not have this poison in their bodies because of their menstrual flow, which is the parallel change Eve's body underwent after the first sin. Therefore, it is the womb that has to neutralize poisonous semen. In this way, women's bodies have the capacity to nullify men's reproductive toxicity resulting from Adam's fall.

Women as Complete Beings

Hildegard's positive depiction of the female body is supported by her appreciation of the physical body of the human being that was created by God with natural elements. Hildegard's relationship between microcosm and macrocosm is apparent in many places in *Cause et cure*. As Adam's body was created from the elements, so too was God's whole creation, and just as the cosmos contains four elements, so does the human body:

> Just as they hold the world together, the elements are the framework of the human body. Their streaming forth and their functions so divide themselves within a person, that a person is held together; just as, poured through the world, they busy themselves. Fire, air, water and earth are in a person, and from them a person is composed. From fire a person has heat, from air, breath, from water, blood, and from earth a person has flesh.[3]

After this assertion, Hildegard continues her discussion of this analogy by detailing the various symptoms and diseases that people may acquire if the

3 In modifying the translation of this passage, I intentionally used "a person" instead of "he" to reflect gender neutrality, which aligns with contemporary translation practices and acknowledges modern understandings of gender inclusivity. Modified from Hildegard of Bingen, *Causes and Cures*, trans. Throop, 42. "Nunc autem, ut supradictum est, quemadmodum elementa mundum simul continent, sic etiam elementa compago corporis hominis sunt, atque effusio et officia eorum ita se diuidunt per hominem, ut insimul contineatur, uelut etiam per mundum effusa sunt et operantur. Ignis enim, aer, aqua et terra in homine sunt et ex hiis constat. Nam ex igne habet calorem, ex aere alitum, ex aqua sanguinem et ex terra carnem." Hildegard of Bingen, *Beate Hildegardis Cause et cure*, ed. Moulinier and Berndt, bk. 2, §97, p. 83.

elements in their bodies, based on the four elements of the world, fall out of balance. The key to staying healthy is maintaining the proper proportions of the bodily humours. People become ill when this balance collapses.[4] However, the correct proportion of the four humours can be different for each person, as expressed in the medical theory of the four temperaments. A person's specific temperament is determined according to which humour is dominant within them. This medical belief prevails among ancient and medieval medical theorists; Hildegard, however, is interesting because she distinguishes women's four temperaments from men's.

Hildegard presents four types of temperament in women after explaining the same four types in men: sanguine, phlegmatic, choleric, and melancholic. Just like men, women have variable bodily humours that determine the degree to which they have different temperamental qualities. In this perspective, even strength of sexual desire (which was often represented elsewhere in medieval writing as uniformly strong and uncontrollable in all women) is different in each woman. Not all women are filled with lust, and not all women desire men equally. Certainly, some women may want sex and need men; however, others do not. In Hildegard's writings, women tend not to fall into one stereotypical type; where males are variable, women are variable, too. Here she describes the sanguine temperament in women:

> These [sanguine] women have a clear, white face and are in the embrace of love. They are loveable and exacting in their skills. They are continent in mind and suffer moderately flowing blood in their streams of menstruation. The vessel of their womb is strongly positioned for child-bearing, whence they are fertile and able to receive the male semen. Nevertheless they do not produce many children. If they are without husbands, and do not give birth to offspring, they easily ail in their body.[5]

---

4 Hildegard of Bingen, *Causes and Cures*, trans. Throop, 48. "Quod si praedicti humores rectum ordinem suum et iustam mensuram, ut praefactum est, in homine seruant, ille in quiete et sanitate corporis est, si autem sibi inuicem repugnauerint, debilem et infirmum, ut prescriptum est, faciunt." Hildegard of Bingen, *Beate Hildegardis Cause et cure*, ed. Moulinier and Berndt, bk. 2, §122, p. 91.

5 Hildegard of Bingen, *Causes and Cures*, trans. Throop, 72. "Et iste claram et albam faciem habent at in amplexione amoris sunt et amabiles atque in artibus subtiles et per se ipsas in animo suo continentes et modice effluentem sanguinem in riuulis menstrui temporis patiuntur, atque uasculum matricis earum fortiter positum est ad pariendum, unde etiam fecunde sunt et uirile semen concipere possunt. Sed tamen plurimos pueros non generant, et si iste absque maritis sunt, ita quod prolem non pariunt, facile dolent in corpore." Hildegard of Bingen, *Beate Hildegardis Cause et cure*, ed. Moulinier and Berndt, bk. 2, §172, p. 126.

Judging from this passage, we can infer that sanguine women may have relatively strong sexual desires for men, since they are happy when they have husbands. The sanguine woman's menstruation is not severe, and her womb is particularly suitable for reproduction, so it seems that these women are the best at having babies. We might say that the sanguine woman benefits from being a wife and mother rather than an ascetic practitioner.

Like sanguine women, phlegmatic women are also described as suitable for reproduction. In the case of the phlegmatic woman, according to Hildegard, childbirth and a sexual life are much desired and encouraged. These women's strong yearning for a sexual life is stated up front in *Cause et cure.* In order to support her characterization of the phlegmatic woman's strong sexual drive and desire to reproduce, Hildegard lists this woman's physical and social characteristics: wide veins, a strongly placed womb, and popularity among men.

> They [phlegmatic women] have a stern face of swarthy complexion. Vigorous, useful, with a somewhat virile mind, they sustain neither too small nor too great, but moderately flowing, streams of blood in their menstrual period. Since they have large veins, they are very fecund for offspring and easily conceive. Their womb and all the internal organs are strongly positioned. They attract men and lead them behind them, and men love them. If they wish to keep themselves from men, they are able to refrain from joining with them, which debilitates them a little, but not much. If they avoid joining with men, they become hard to deal with and serious in their behavior; if they are with men, and refuse to hold themselves back from union, they become incontinent and overflow with lust, just like men.[6]

In this view, just like sanguine women, or even more so, phlegmatic women enjoy their sexual lives. They are happy with children and can even become sick if they cannot have intercourse with men, and men like them in return. Certainly, they may experience difficulties if they choose the monastic life.

---

6 Hildegard of Bingen, *Causes and Cures*, trans. Throop, 72–73. "Et seueram faciem et subnigri coloris habent et strenue et utiles sunt ac aliquantum uirilem animum tenent, atque nec nimis parum nec nimis multum, sed moderate effluentes riuulos sanguinis in menstruo tempore sustinent. Et quoniam grossas uenas habent, plurimum fecunde sunt in prole et facile concipiunt, quia etiam matrix et omnia uiscera earum fortiter posita sunt. Sed uiros sibi attrahunt et eos post se ducunt, et ideo uiri eas amant. Quod si a uiris se continere uolunt, se continere a coniunctione eorum possunt, nec inde multum quamuis parum debilitantur. Sed tamen, si uiros in coniunctione deuitauerint, difficiles et graues in moribus suis erunt, si autem cum uiris fuerint, ita quod se a coniunctione eorum continere noluerint, incontinentes et superflue secundum uiros in libidine erunt." Hildegard of Bingen, *Beate Hildegardis Cause et cure*, ed. Moulinier and Berndt, bk. 2, §173, pp. 126–27.

These women are too fertile to reject husbands and sexual activity; abstinence can make them sick. Also, phlegmatic women are good at giving birth. Like sanguine women, they have wombs that are securely positioned in their bodies. What is more notable, phlegmatic women can deliver a number of children. They release a moderate amount of blood during menstruation. It is interesting that phlegmatic women are desired by men even though they have "manly" souls. In every sense, they seem very apt for reproduction.

Choleric women do not seem unhappy with their sexual lives; however, their mode of behaviour is slightly different in that men tend to avoid these women, although men love them, too. After discussing their physical characteristics, Hildegard turns to the topic of choleric women's love lives:

> They [choleric women] are shown respect by men, and are feared. They suffer in menstruation with very much blood. Their womb is strongly positioned, and they are fertile. Men love their ways, but avoid them a bit. These women do not draw men behind them, alluring them. If they are joined to husbands, they are chaste and observe wifely fidelity. With husbands, they are physically healthy, but if they lack them, they will feel pain in their body, and they will be weak, as much from not knowing to whom they might show womanly fidelity, as from the fact they do not have husbands. If the flows of the menstrual period ease before the due time, they will easily be paralytic and they will be enervated and infirm in their humors, or they will feel pain in their liver, or easily incur the black tumor of *dragunculus*, or their breasts swell up from cancer.[7]

Choleric women have a bit of a complicated character. Men generally love these women, but they are reluctant to be near them, since choleric women do not let men chase after them, unlike phlegmatic women, who seem to easily draw men to them. However, once choleric women are married, Hildegard states that they are loyal to their husbands. In addition, choleric

7 Hildegard of Bingen, *Causes and Cures*, trans. Throop, 73. "Et eis reuerentia ab hominibus exhibetur, et timentur. Sed plurimum sanguinem in menstruis patiuntur, et matrix in eis fortiter posita est, ac fecunde sunt. Et uiri mores earum amant, sed tamen eas aliquantum deuitando fugiunt, quoniam ipse illos alliciendo illos post se non trahunt. Quod si in coniuncione maritorum sunt, caste sunt et fidem uxorum illis seruant atque cum eis sane sunt in corpore, et si maritis caruerint, dolebunt in corpore et debiles erunt tam de hoc, quod nesciunt, cui homini femineam fidem seruare possint, quam de hoc, quod maritos non habent. Et si fluenta menstrui temporis prius, quam iustum sit, in eis cessauerint, facile paralitice erunt et in humoribus suis diffluunt, ita quod in eisdem humoribus suis infirme erunt aut quod in iecore dolebunt aut quod etiam facile nigrum tumorem dragunculi incurrunt aut quod ubera earum de cancro ingrossantur." Hildegard of Bingen, *Beate Hildegardis Cause et cure*, ed. Moulinier and Berndt, bk. 2, §174, pp. 127–28.

women have active sexual lives, and they are healthier when they have husbands. When they are not with men, their bodily systems develop issues that weaken them.

On the other hand, choleric women do not seem to benefit much from reproduction. While Hildegard explains that sanguine and phlegmatic women may have many or few children, she barely discusses reproduction in choleric women, emphasizing instead that choleric women might experience a good deal of pain and copious bleeding during menstruation. However, the good thing about the choleric woman's reproductive system is that her womb is securely positioned in her body, and she has minimal reproductive health issues.

In drawing such distinctions, Hildegard introduces the idea that qualities of temperament vary greatly among women. Sanguine and choleric women have similarities in that both types of women need men in order to remain healthy. They are likely to fall ill if they lack husbands. They are good at having babies, as their wombs are securely placed. But their reproductive strengths also suggest that they may not be well suited for ascetic life, in which women have to avoid all men but Jesus.

At the same time, there are some interesting women who do not need men according to Hildegard's physiology. Or rather, they are healthier when they avoid men. These are the melancholic women. The melancholic woman is different from the other female temperament types, which have strong sexual appetites or a high degree of attractiveness to men. According to Hildegard, melancholic women tend to be busy with their own pursuits and less interested in men. They are easily lost in thought and easily tired. These women are not only indifferent to men but are also ignored by men in return. Furthermore, their bodily characteristics are not the most suitable for conceiving and delivering babies.

> They [melancholic women] suffer very much blood in their menstrual period, and are sterile, since they have a weak, fragile womb. Whence they are not able to receive, retain, or warm the man's semen. They are healthier, stronger, and happier without husbands than with them since, if they are with husbands, they are enfeebled. Men turn away from them and flee them because they do not address men affably, and they love men very little. If these women at any time have delectation of the flesh, it quickly ceases.[8]

8 Hildegard of Bingen, *Causes and Cures*, trans. Throop, 73. "Sed et plurimum sanguinem in menstruo tempore patiuntur et steriles sunt, quia debilem et fragilem matricem habent. Vnde semen uiri nec concipere nec retinere nec calefacere possunt, et ideo etiam saniores, fortiores et letiores sunt absque maritis quam cum eis,

These women are not well suited for reproduction, which is the primary duty of women in medieval society outside the monastery. Hildegard argues that many melancholic women can be infertile. It is not their fault, nor is it unnatural. Rather, it is the natural result of their physical disposition and character given by God. These women do not have strong wombs like sanguine and choleric women. Also, melancholic women do not need men as much as sanguine or choleric women. Melancholic women are not happy when men are around them, because they do not want to talk to them, and they become rather sick if they have husbands. Even when melancholic women get a taste of carnal pleasure, they do not enjoy it for long. Hildegard concludes that they are not well suited to conceiving and having babies in general, although there is one exception: even melancholic women can be happy with sanguine men. They can have a happy marriage, as they have natures that correspond and balance each other's temperaments. Otherwise, melancholic women are better off living alone.

Even though Hildegard does not make this explicit, she implies that melancholic women are well adapted to remaining virgins and pursuing a religious life. Since they do not have strong sexual impulses, and these diminish rather quickly when they appear, they have fewer issues with monastic life than sanguine or choleric women, who are known for their inclination towards men. Even better, men do not care much for melancholic women in return. These women could be understood as less dangerous for males in monasteries, since there is less of a chance that they will seem attractive to religious men or lead them to sin. Indeed, as Hildegard comments elsewhere, licentiousness is a problem of individual temperament, not gender-specific.[9] This understanding is contrary to ancient and medieval male writ-

---

quoniam, si cum maritis fuerint, debiles reddentur. Sed uiri ab eis declinant et eas fugiunt, quia ipsae uiros affabiliter non allocuntur, et quoniam uiros modice diligunt. Et si iste ad horam aliquam delectationem carnis habuerint, cito tamen in eis deficit." Hildegard of Bingen, *Beate Hildegardis Cause et cure*, ed. Moulinier and Berndt, bk. 2, §175, p. 128.

9 "Other people, unrestrained in lust, neither have, nor seek to have, continence. Their blood is often inordinately shaken; like a pot placed on a fire which, getting neither completely hot nor completely cool, holds in filthy matter, without powers enough to throw it off." Hildegard of Bingen, *Causes and Cures*, trans. Throop, 130. "Sunt et alii quidam homines de libedine incontinentes, ita quod nec continentiam habent nec eam habere querunt, unde sanguis eorum sepe et inordinate concutitur, uelut olla ad ignem posita, que nec ex toto feruet nec ex toto frigida est, et sic sordes in se retinet, quia tantas uires in se non habet, quod eas eiciat." Hildegard of Bingen, *Beate Hildegardis Cause et cure*, ed. Moulinier and Berndt, bk. 2, §343, p. 200.

ers' view that women were so incomplete that they might need intercourse with men to stay healthy. For example, the popular gynaecological book *De secretis mulierum* falsely cites Galen to explain that a woman's mysterious symptoms were caused by a lack of sexual activity with men.[10]

Clearly, Hildegard does not judge women's nature as though it had one singular characteristic, namely, strong sexuality; instead, she introduces different types of women according to their physiological temperaments and psychological complexions. Just as with men, the intensity of their sexual desire varies, depending on their temperaments. Though she refers to herself as "weak" and "inferior," she writes in a way that shows that women are not any less complex than men, and because they have very different qualities among themselves, they cannot be understood as comprising a single category of licentious, naive, and ill-natured beings.[11] Nor can women simply be reduced to one half of the Aristotelian dualistic physiology that casts them as cold and passive.[12] Just like men, some women are more sexual than others. Some are well suited for religious and solitary lives, while others are better suited for various social activities, childbirth, and family life. Women are not equally filled with sexual desire, nor equally licentious, nor equally born to have children. Her account of women's differing temperaments indicates Hildegard's own interest in and dedication to the study of women's physiology. Rather than assigning one

---

10 "The greater doctor Galen tells about a certain woman who was suffering a suffocation of the womb so serious that it prevented her from talking, and she fell down as if she were dead, with no sign of life...Galen then came on the scene, considered the cause, and freed the woman from this illness. This sickness happens in women because they are full of corrupt and poisonous menses, and therefore it is good that these women, whether young or old, often use men, so that this matter might be expelled. This is especially helpful in young women, because they are full of humidity." Pseudo-Albertus Magnus, *Women's Secrets*, trans. Lemay, 132. "Galenus enim magnus in medicina, narrat de quadam muliere, suffocationem matricis patiente, quòd illa causa patiebatur tantum quod non potuit loqui, & cecideit ac si mortua esset, quia nullum signum vitae habuit, ...Galenus autem superueniẽs, causam considerauit, & mulierem à passione illa liberauit. Hęc enim aegritudo contingit in mulieribus ex eo que abundat in eis menstruũ corrumptum & venenosum. Et ideo bonum est quòd tales mulieres, quaecunque fuerint, siue iuuenes, sine antiquae, saepe viris vtantur, vt materia talis expellatur. Et expedit iuuenibus, quia in eis abundant humidum. Pseudo-Albertus Magnus, *De secretis mulierum*, 123–24.

11 Relying in part on arguments from Hildegard, Margaret Miles criticizes male-centred history that builds up a singular image of women. Miles, *Carnal Knowing*, 172.

12 Cadden, "It Takes All Kinds," 155.

nature or one duty to women, she suggests that women, like men, have different physical and psychological characteristics that make them suited for different possible ways of living.

Menstruation as Punishment

In canon law compilations and commentaries, there was debate about whether women should be allowed in church during menstruation or after delivering a child. Hildegard is different from other canonists before her in that she does not particularly distinguish between men and women in ritual purity. Unlike Gratian, Rufinus, and Paucapalea, Hildegard applies one criterion to both women's and men's bodies—whether they are whole or not. Moreover, Hildegard is interesting because her views are supported by her medical accounts, which we have seen in *Cause et cure*. In her eyes, just as there is no physical reason to see menstruation as polluting, there is no reason to forbid menstruating women from entering the church in *Scivias*. Even when defloration and childbirth seem to justify reading the body as corrupt, Hildegard finds a physical basis for comparing such women's broken bodies to the wounds of men. This distinguishes her views from those of Gratian and Gregory, who allowed women's entrance into the church only because women had already been punished by childbirth despite their "fleshly delight" and Eve's transgression.[13] Therefore, it is meaningful that even when Hildegard forbade women from entering the church after childbirth, she did not attribute her reasoning to women's sinful or physical nature.

Gratian, a contemporary of Hildegard, took menstruating and postpartum women's side on this issue. Like Hildegard, Gratian argues that men should not approach menstruating women sexually, and that women should not stop nursing their own babies just because they want to have intercourse with their husbands again. Here, he does not give a specific reason for this prohibition, such as women's pain or their polluting nature, other than Leviticus: "For the sacred law [Lev. 20:18] inflicted death on a man who approached a menstruating woman." However, following Gregory the Great, Gratian still argues that menstruating women should be permitted to enter

13 "If a woman, in the very hour she gives birth, enters a church to give thanks, she incurs no burden of sin for there is fault in fleshly delight, not in pain...So then, if we were to forbid a woman who has given birth from entering a church, we would be classing her very punishment as a fault." Gratian, *Treatise on Laws*, trans. Gordley, dist. 5, chap. 2, p. 17.

the church.[14] Gregory argued that if these women were forbidden to enter the church, it was like punishing them twice, considering that they already suffer from the punishment of Eve.[15] Moreover, according to Gratian's understanding of Gregory, the church already had an example in the woman with bleeding issues from the Gospel who was healed by touching Jesus' garment. Jesus was not angry with her; rather, he complimented her courage.

On the other hand, a few theologians did not show mercy to women during menstruation or the postpartum period. Rufinus, a twelfth-century commentator on Gratian who was also an influential figure in the later tradition of canon law,[16] disagrees with Gratian and Gregory on whether postpartum women could enter the church. His commentary on the *Decretum* relies more on the old purity laws and Theodore's *Penitentials* to support his position against permitting women entrance into the church right after childbirth.[17] Rufinus refers to Julius Solinus on the harmful effects of menstrual

14 "Nevertheless, a woman undergoing the usual period of menstruation should not be prohibited from entering a church since fault ought not to be imputed to an excrescence of nature. Thus, it is unjust that, on account of what is suffered unwillingly, they be deprived of entrance into a church. For we know that the woman who suffered from the issue of blood, coming up behind the Lord, touched the hem of his garment and was immediately freed from her infirmity [Matt. 9:20–23]. . . . And later: If, then, it was proper that the woman presumed to touch the Lord's garment in her illness, why should what was granted to one infirm person not be conceded to all women who endure a similar infirmity due to a natural debility?" Gratian, *Treatise on Laws*, trans. Gordley, dist. 5, chap. 2, p. 18.

15 On the other hand, Gregory still considered menstruation as a defect, even though menstruating women could enter the church if they really wanted to. "For the menstruous habit in women is no sin, seeing that it occurs naturally; yet still that nature itself has been so vitiated as to be seen to be polluted even without the intention of the will is a defect that comes of sin, whereby human nature may perceive what through judgment it has come to be, so that man who voluntarily committed sin may bear the guilt of sin involuntarily. And so females, when they consider themselves as being in their habit of sickness, if they presume not to approach the sacrament of the body and blood of the Lord, are to be commended for their right consideration." Gregory the Great, *Registrum epistolarum*, trans. Barmby, bk. 11, ep. 64.

16 Raming, *History of Women and Ordination*, 2:80.

17 "Dicitur autem in hac dist. ex auctoritate Gregorii [cap. II, III] quod mulier enixa mox licite potest intrare ecclesiam, ut puer natus statim baptizari; similiter etiam menstruata. Tamen ab utriusque concubitu, dum et illa est in purgatione et ista in profluvio sanguinis, viri se continere debent. Illud de enixa vero muliere hodie evacuatum est propter ecclesie contrariam consuetudinem et maxime propter illud ex penitentiali Theodori, quod est in Brocard. lib. XIX., capitulo (141), 'Mulier que intrat ecclesiam ante mundum sanguinem post partum, si masculum genuerit, XXXIII

blood.[18] Furthermore, he also saw women's pregnancy as polluting because "every unformed foetus displeases God," meaning the female reproductive processes are harmful in general.[19]

These debates reveal a negative attitude in the theology of Hildegard's time towards women during or immediately after the loss of blood, showing that Hildegard was on the cutting edge of issues regarding whether women should be permitted to enter the church during menstruation and after childbirth. The ancient belief in ritual impurity to see menstruation as polluting and dangerous lingered in medieval society. Even when theologians granted entrance to the church to menstruating women, they could still blame women's bodies for polluting men, as Gratian's pupil Paucapalea did, citing the *Penitentials* of Theodore in his argument.[20] Even when women

dies' – a die octava i. e. circumcisionis; 'si feminam, LXVI' – post quartam decimam diem, quando convenientibus amicis nomen puelle imponebatur – ab ingressu ecclesie abstineat." Rufinus, *Summa decretorum*, ed. Singer, dist. 5, p. 16.

18 "Menstruata autem mulier dicitur a menstruis, i. e. a profluvio sanguinis, quod per menses singulos mulier perfert; hec etiam muliebria nuncupantur. Adeo autem execrabilis et immundus est sanguis ille, sicut ait Iulius Solinus in libro de mirabilibus mundi, ut eius contactu fruges non germinent, arescant arbusta, moriantur herbe, amittant arbores fetus, nigrescant era, si canes inde ederint in rabiem efferantur. Non autem solum propter ipsam immunditiam sanguinis a menstruata arcenda est voluptas, sed etiam ne vitiosus fetus ex illo coitu nascatur; tunc enim testante Ieronymo concepti fetus vitium seminis contrahunt, ita ut leprosi et elefantici ex hac corruptione nascantur et feda corpora in utroque sexu parvitate vel deformitate membrorum appareant; sanies enim corrupta degenerat." Rufinus, *Summa decretorum*, ed. Singer, dist. 5, pp. 16–17.

19 "Quo spatio arcetur mulier ab ingressu templi tamquam immunda, ut per hoc innuatur quod omnis fetus informis displicet Deo; sola enim formosa placent Deo – unde sponsus ad sponsam dicit: Amica mea, formosa mea. Sed iuxta hanc considerationem ab introitu templi prohiberi debuerat, cum fetus in utero informis erat, non post partum, cum iam sit formatus et natus. Quod tamen fit, eo quod nescitur, quo tempore concipiatur, cum in utero illud secretum agitur, ideoque quod [fieri] non potuit eo tempore propter ignorantiam fit eo tempore, quo potest, cum iam scitur: ut scil. post partum mulier illud suppleat, quod secundum ordinem nature ante partum fieri debuerat." Rufinus, *Summa decretorum*, ed. Singer, dist. 5, p. 17.

20 "Menstrua dicitur supervacuus mulieris sanguis. Dicta vero menstrua a lunaria luminis circuito a quo hoc solet evenire profluvium. Luna enim graece mene dicitur. Haec et muliebria nuncupantur. Nam solum mulier menstruale animal est, cuius contactu sanguinis fruges non germinant, acescunt musta, moriuntur herbae, amittunt arbores fructus, ferrum rubigo corrumpit, nigrescunt aera; si canes inde ederint in rabiem efferuntur. Et sciendum est, quod, ut dicit beatus Gregorius: Si mulier hora eadem etc. Sed in poenitentiali Theodori contra legitur, ut si mulier ante praefinitum tempus praesumpserit ecclesiam intrare, tot dies in pane et aqua

were admitted into the church after childbirth, they were allowed to enter only under certain conditions, such as the women's humility and prayer. This implies that women's bodily characteristics were still seen as going against the church's teaching—as something that required penance. Even when male theologians such as Gratian allowed women to enter the church during their periods or after delivering a child, they were not entirely free of negative views towards menstruating or postpartum bodies. According to male theologians, women were allowed into the church "despite" their bodily defects.

In Hildegard's discourse on what women should or should not do, she often omits discussion of pollution, which sharply distinguishes her from male theologians. Even when Hildegard explains why menstruating women should not have intercourse, it is not about pollution but about their physical distress. She argues, in God's voice, that menstruating women should not have intercourse with men—not because they are polluting but because they are already in pain. As women are not polluting but in pain, it is not fair if they are not allowed in church, especially during the time when women need care.[21] Women with their periods should keep themselves "in hidden knowledge,"[22] but this does not mean that they should be prevented from entering the church. A woman's church visit, guaranteed by her faith, is for salvation.

While Hildegard, like Gratian, does not see menstruation as a sufficient reason to keep women from church, she differs from him in viewing childbirth as a valid reason for keeping women away from church. Her view is unique. For example, Gratian, following Gregory, sees no reason to keep women from giving thanks in church after a successful childbirth. Hilde-

---

poeniteat, quot ecclesia carere debuerat. Solutio. Beatus Greg, illam dicit in hoc non peccare, quae gratias actura humiliter ecclesiam ingreditur. Theodore vero de ea dicit, quae non causa orationis sed alia qualibet necessitate ducta temere ingreditur. Sic et menstrua orationis causa non prohibetur ecclesiam ingredi." Paucapalea, *Summa*, ed. von Schulte, dist. 5, 11. Translated in Raming, *History of Women and Ordination*, 2:101n45.

21 Hildegard of Bingen, *Scivias*, trans. Hart and Bishop, 83. "Sed hoc tempus doloris in muliere non abicio, quoniam illud Euae dedi quando in gustu pomi peccatum concepit, unde et mulier in hoc eodem tempore in magna medicina misericordiae habenda est." Hildegard of Bingen, *Scivias*, ed. Führkötter and Carelvaris, pt. 1, bk. 2, chap. 20, p. 27.

22 Hildegard of Bingen, *Scivias*, trans. Hart and Bishop, 83. "Ipsa etiam se continente in absconso disciplinae, non autem ita ut ab incessu templi mei se contineat." Hildegard of Bingen, *Scivias*, ed. Führkötter and Carelvaris, pt. 1, bk. 2, chap. 20, p. 27.

gard does. Her reason in God's voice for this has to do with bodily wholeness: whether women undergo any processes which might bring about serious injury. It does not specifically concern women's issues. As we have seen in her *Cause et cure*, menstruation simply takes advantage of natural openings in the womb to rid the body of surplus fluids; it does not break a woman's body apart. Childbirth, however, is a more serious event for Hildegard, as it involves a rupture of a woman's wholeness.

In either case, Hildegard does not focus on the polluted or polluting nature of the woman's body in reproductive processes. In particular, menstruation is far from being a matter of pollution, because it does not rupture or wound the female body. Hildegard suggests that a woman's body has a pathway that allows air to enter, which benefits the release of menstrual blood and allows a baby to breathe when needed.[23] When God opened Eve's body after she ate the forbidden fruit, God also opened the bodies of her female descendants. Therefore, menstruation became a routine part of the earthly existence of women. This accounts for why, except when they are pregnant, women are bound to menstruate monthly. Hildegard, like other medieval theologians, understands this "small portion of the pain of childbirth"[24] as a part of women's penance; however, she does not portray the bodies of menstruating women as dangerous to men but rather emphasizes women's need for nurturing tenderness in times of menstruation or pregnancy.

However, postpartum women are different because their bodies have such "open" wounds that they should not be allowed in church. Yet, this is not because they are women and have to go through reproductive processes. The reason is physical and not limited to women. Hildegard says that a broken body could be a pollution, but this is not exclusive to women. Pollution from a broken body can happen to men.[25] Hildegard elaborates by referring

---

23 While women were already weak and fragile when they were created by God, a woman's openness increases during menstruation and pregnancy so that the flow of blood and air can come in and go out. For example, a woman's skull is divided, and her skin is thin, enabling these flows. Newman, *Sister of Wisdom*, 128–29.

24 Hildegard of Bingen, *Scivias*, trans. Hart and Bishop, 83. "Portionem scilicet doloris partus sui tangens." Hildegard of Bingen, *Scivias*, ed. Führkötter and Carelvaris, pt. 1, bk. 2, chap. 20, p. 27.

25 Hildegard of Bingen, *Scivias*, trans. Hart and Bishop, 83. "Sed et mulier cum prolem pepererit fractis occultis membris suis templum meum nonnisi secundum legem per me sibi datam ingrediatur, quatenus sancta sacramenta eiusdem templi mei ab omni pollutione et dolore uiri ac mulieris inuiolabilia sint; quia Filium meum purissima Virgo genuit, quae integra absque ullo uulnere peccati fuit. Locus enim,

to Leviticus, which says that a man with wounds is also prohibited from entering a holy place. The wounds that women receive from childbirth and that men receive from "the impact of a blow"[26] are treated in the same way. This openness from childbirth is not the same, however, as the openness that enables the menstrual flow in the woman's body. The former is more like a rupture.

For Hildegard, a rupture matters. She goes on to explain the reason why a person with an open wound is not allowed in church, which is to preserve the wholeness of the Ecclesia; for Hildegard, as she repeatedly emphasizes, this wholeness is analogous to virginity and the wholeness of the Virgin Mary. A rupture of the physical body, which Hildegard traces all the way back to the broken body of Abel slaughtered by Cain,[27] meant a schism of the Church, like the schism that Hildegard faced in her time.[28] This interpretation is valid because the human being's physical body is not only analogically but literally the temple of God. Just as the temple of God should not be divided, the ruptured human body should be kept away from the healthy church.

---

qui in honorem eiusdem Vnigeniti mei consecratus est, integer ab omni corruptione liuoris ac uulneris esse debet; quoniam idem Vnigenitus meus integritatem uirginei partus in se nouit. Vnde et mulier quae integritatem uirginitatis suae cum uiro corrumpit, in liuore plagae suae qua corrupta est ab ingressu templi mei se contineat, usque dum plaga uulneris ipsius sanetur secundum quod ecclesiastica disciplina ipsi de eadem causa certissime demonstrat." Hildegard of Bingen, *Scivias*, ed. Führkötter and Carelvaris, pt. 1, bk. 2, chap. 21, p. 28.

26 Hildegard of Bingen, *Scivias*, trans. Hart and Bishop, 83. "Uir (apertis uulneribus si integritas membrorum ipsius in tactu percussionis diuisa est) templum meum nisi cum timore magnae necessitatis non intrabit ne uioletur." Hildegard of Bingen, *Scivias*, ed. Führkötter and Carelvaris, pt. 1, bk. 2, chap. 20, p. 27.

27 Hildegard of Bingen, *Scivias*, trans. Hart and Bishop, 83. "Sicut integra membra Abel, qui templum Dei fuit, Cain frater suus crudeliter fregit." Hildegard of Bingen, *Scivias*, ed. Führkötter and Carelvaris, pt. 1, bk. 2, chap. 20, p. 27.

28 After her death, it seems that Hildegard's writings on schism were understood as authoritative precedents to be consulted for advice in later crises. For example, Pierre d'Ailly (1350/1351–1420), a famous theologian, consulted Hildegard of Bingen's writings as prophecies about the Great Schism, although Laura Ackerman Smoller argues that it is hard to determine how much she impacted him. Smoller, *History, Prophecy, and the Stars*, 97. Renate Blumenfeld-Kosinski suggests that Hildegard was seen as a major prophet, read more importantly after her lifetime, especially during the time of the Great Schism. Blumenfeld-Kosinski, "Visions and Schism Politics," 173–87.

And even for Hildegard, deflowering and childbirth are not very different from the physical bruises and wounds of men. Hildegard sees them as representing the same level of loss of bodily integrity; wounds are thus treated as corruptions. As she writes: "Therefore, let a woman who breaks the wholeness of her virginity with a man also refrain from entering My Temple while injured by the bruise of her corruption, until the injury of that wound is healed."[29] Hildegard did not treat women's bodies after intercourse and childbirth as polluted or polluting because they were undergoing uniquely *feminine* processes; rather, her prohibitions are based on the commonalities between men and women. Corruption from bruises could happen to anyone. And once their wounds were healed, whether earned through sexual activity or physical combat, both men and women needed to re-establish contact with the community of the faithful and could enter churches to do so. From this perspective, women's bodily processes were no more polluting than men's. In fact, in the context of its necessity as a part of the perpetuation of humankind, sexual intercourse was not dirty. Hildegard thus focuses on the wounding nature of deflowering, without making intercourse itself problematic. For Hildegard, the most important factor in deciding whether someone should be accepted into the church was whether their bodies were wounded or whole.

On a related note, it is also interesting that Hildegard juxtaposes Eve and Cain in explaining whether or not women should be allowed to go to church during menstruation or after childbirth. In some sense, Eve—who introduced original sin and therefore death, and was punished with painful childbirth—and Cain—who committed homicide for the first time, and therefore breached the temple of the body and threatened the wholeness of the church—could be considered similar insofar as they were the first sinners, and thus prompted the association of certain bodily states in men and women with parallel penances. As these passages of Hildegard's *Scivias* show, she promotes ideas that tend to equalize male and female problems; she does not emphasize the polluting or inferior nature of the female body when she (in God's voice) allows menstruating women to enter the church.

29 Hildegard of Bingen, *Scivias*, trans. Hart and Bishop, 83. "Vnde et mulier quae integritatem uirginitatis suae cum uiro corrumpit, in liuore plagae suae qua corrupta est ab ingressu templi mei se contineat, usque dum plaga uulneris ipsius sanetur." Hildegard of Bingen, *Scivias*, ed. Führkötter and Carelvaris, pt. 1, bk. 2, chap. 21, p. 28.

Menstruation as Purgative

Hildegard states that women's menstruation functions to cleanse their bodies by expelling unnecessary blood and humours. However, Hildegard goes further than her contemporaries by suggesting that women's blood also functions to detoxify men's semen, which changed after Adam's transgression; in describing the process of emitting seed and conception, she reverses the normal polarity of heat and cold that characterized women and men in medieval physiology. Describing the condition of the parents' bodies at conception, she writes:

> These all create a tempest, from their excessive superfluity. From the blood, they bring forth a poisonous foam, which is semen. When it falls upon its place, the blood of the mother joins with it, from which it will be bloody. Conception of a human being arises from pleasure, which the serpent, in the first fruit, blew into the human; the man's blood is spurred on by pleasure. That blood sends cold foam into the woman; the heat of the maternal flesh coagulates it, spreading it out into a bloody form. The foam, remaining in the heat, soon grows dense, to the stature of a small human being, from the sweat of dry foods of the mother; until the writing of the creator, which formed the human being, overlays a consistent density on the human stature; just as a workman forms a tall vessel.[30]

In this passage, it is not women's menstrual material but men's semen which is toxic. This idea of poison in the semen is repeated:

> In Adam's transgression, the strength in the male's genital member changed into a poisonous foam, and the female's blood changed to a contrary effusion. Because men's flesh was made from earth, his blood has semen of a strong and correct nature. A woman's blood is also of a correct nature. Because she is weak and tender she does not have semen, but emits merely a tiny, watery foam, since she is not of both earth and flesh, as a male, but was taken only from the flesh of the male. And so she is weak and fragile and

30 Hildegard of Bingen, *Causes and Cures*, trans. Throop, 51. "Et hec omnia de nimietate superfluitatis quasi tempestatem faciunt et de sanguine uenenosam spumam, quod semen est, educunt, quod, cum in locum suum cadit, sanguis mulieris illi se coniungit, et ex hoc sanguineum erit. Prima enim inceptio hominis per delectationem, quam serpens in pomo primo homini insufflauit, exoritur, quia tunc sanguis uiri ex delectatione concutitur. Vnde et idem sanguis frigidam spumam mulieri inmittit, que ex calore materne carnis coagulatur et in sanguineam formam extenditur; ac eadem spuma in eodem calore sic permanens postmodum a sudore sicci ciborum matris in spissitudinem parue humane stature crescit, quousque scriptura creatoris, que hominem formauit, eandem spissitudinem humane stature totam perfundit, quemadmodum faber elatum uas suum format." Hildegard of Bingen, *Beate Hildegardis Cause et cure*, ed. Moulinier and Berndt, bk. 2, §129, p. 95.

> is the vessel of a man. From the love of the male, her blood is aroused and she sends it, as if a foam, more bloody than white, to the semen of the male.[31]

Hildegard argues that women's wombs have the power to heat men's semen and to neutralize semen's poisonous nature in the complementary process of conception. This view is interesting because traditionally, women's bodies were considered colder than men's. Hildegard also acknowledges this, and she generally follows this Galenic conception of male and female physiology. However, Hildegard emphasizes the complementary relationship between the two sexes to such a degree that she still envisions interactions between women and men during reproductive processes.

> It joins with it and shapes it, making it warm and bloody. After it has fallen into its place, and lain there, it grows cold. It is as if a poisonous foam until fire, that is heat, warms it and until air, that is breath, dries it; and until water, that is liquid, allows pure dampness to enter; and until the earth, that is a membrane, constrains it. And then it will be bloody—not totally blood, but combined with a bit of blood. The four humors, which she[32] draws from the four elements, remain in moderate balance around this semen until, as if flesh, it is coagulated and firmed so that the shape of a human can be configured in it.[33]

---

31 Modified from Hildegard of Bingen, *Causes and Cures*, trans. Throop, 51. "Nam in transgressione Ade fortitudo uiri in genitali membro uersus est in uenenosam spumam, atque mulieris sanguis uersus est in contrariam effusionem. De forti enim et de recta natura uiri sanguis eius semen habet, quia de terra caro factus est. Sed de recta natura mulieris sanguis eius, quia debilis et tenuis est, semen non habet, sed tantum tenuem et paruam spumam emittit, quoniam de duobus modis terre et carnis non est ut uir, sed tantum de carne uiri sumpta est; et ideo debilis et fragilis est et uas uiri est. Et de amore uiri sanguis eius concutitur et uelut spumam, sed magis sanguineam quam albam, ad semen uiri emittit." Hildegard of Bingen, *Beate Hildegardis Cause et cure*, ed. Moulinier and Berndt, bk. 1, §129, pp. 95–96.

32 Throop identified the subject as "he" in her translation, but I argue that the subject should be "she" rather than "he" because it is the mother who draws on the four elements and uses them to strengthen the foetus.

33 Modified from Hildegard of Bingen, *Causes and Cures*, trans. Throop, 51–52. "Que se illi coniungit et que illud calidum et sanguineum facit et confortat. Nam postquam in locum suum ceciderit et iacuerit, frigescit. Et tam diu quasi uenenosa spuma est, usque dum ignis, uidelicet calor, illud calefacit, et dum aer, uidelicet spiramen, illud exsiccat, et dum aqua, scilicet fluor, illi puram humiditatem admittit, et usque dum terra, scilicet cutecula, illud constringit. Et tunc sic erit sanguineum, id est non totum sanguis, sed aliquantulum sanguine permixtum. Et quatuor humores, quos homo a quatuor elementis trahit, ita circa idem semen moderate et temperate manent, usque dum quasi caro coaguletur et confirmetur, ita quod forma hominis in eo figurari potest." Hildegard of Bingen, *Beate Hildegardis Cause et cure*, ed. Moulinier and Berndt, bk. 2, §129, p. 96.

Men have to heat women's bodies with their love, and women's foam, the female version of semen, will then warm men's semen. Rather than fixing the binary nature of women and men, Hildegard values the fact that women and men exchange qualities in order to reproduce. Both sexes work together because women and men are made to become one flesh; their natures are complementary (in strength and weakness as well as in heat and cold). However, when Hildegard analyzes the actual process of conception, she reverts to this gendered hot–cold polarity. At the moment of conception, it is the woman's womb that is hotter and does the work of warming men's semen, which is colder.

Hildegard's suggestion that men have poisonous semen represents another major departure from Aristotle, Galen, and their medieval followers, who hold that semen is the purest and most distilled form of blood. During the organic process of conception, semen is joined with women's foam, surrounded by women's humours, and heated by the womb in order to grow into a human form.

Because the womb nurtures and strengthens, the mixture of men's semen and women's foam allows the embryo to develop into a child by eliminating semen's dangerous nature. In this sense, the womb provides not only a nutritive but also a purifying environment for babies. Carrying this idea further, it is ultimately the womb that nullifies the result of Adam's sin in God's creation story by re-creation through the Virgin Mary, who conceived Jesus as a part of God's plan to purify the entire human generation; more on the purifying role of female bodies will be discussed in the next chapter. What is important here is that every woman to some extent engages in a purifying process during conception.

By reframing menstruation as a purgative process rather than the cause and result of pollution, Hildegard ties a medical perspective on female physiology to a theological understanding of redemption. Her appreciation of physical flows as divinely intended mechanisms of balance contrasts with her male predecessors and contemporaries who viewed these reproductive processes primarily as manifestations of Eve's curse. This integration of medical and theological perspectives reinterprets the premodern understanding of the womb and women's bodies through a woman's voice.

Chapter 4

RECEIVING THE SPIRIT, FOAM, AND FLUIDS

WHO CONTRIBUTES MORE to making a baby, men or women? Against the prevalent view of her time that men provided the essential elements for creating new life, Hildegard emphasized the complementary relationship between the sexes. She saw reproduction as a collaborative process where neither men nor women could create offspring alone, just as God and human beings were inseparable. While the woman's body is often represented as a passive entity, Hildegard's understanding is quite the opposite: the female body not only receives but also purifies and creates the living. At the same time, it also kindles, nourishes, and develops the reproductive materials. Additionally, the birth of a baby is comparable to God's creation of Eve. Just as God created the first human beings using the four elements and breath, the woman's body uses its four elements and humours and the soul sent from God. The woman's body is optimized for this because it is already acclimated to flow. The foetus's soul flows in through the womb just like God's breath flowed into Eve. The elements of the universe flow and are present in the form of the humours in a woman's body, which nurtures and grows the embryo. These processes occur only within the woman's body.

Women's and Men's Complementary Roles in Intercourse

Hildegard's writings maintain the view that men are stronger and women are subordinated to men.[1] However, a woman's relative weakness is an equal part of a complementary relationship, just like a man's virility. Men are stronger because women are weaker.[2] Eve is a reservoir of the prophetic knowledge that God sent to Adam in his sleep, and she is also the reservoir

1 "The woman is subject to the man in that he sows his seed in her, as he works the earth to make it bear fruit." Hildegard of Bingen, *Scivias*, trans. Hart and Bishop, 84. "Mulier uiro subiecta est in qua ipse semen suum seminet, sicut etiam terram operator ut fructum afferat." Hildegard of Bingen, *Scivias*, ed. Führkötter and Carelvaris, pt. 1, bk. 2, chap. 22, p. 29.

2 Newman also points out the importance of Eve in enabling Adam to become aware of himself, having her as a mirror and reflection. Newman, *Sister of Wisdom*, 94–98.

of future offspring.[3] Hildegard describes women and men as so complementary that they cannot exist without each other.

> Male and female are joined together, therefore, in such a way that each one works through the other. The male would not be called "male" without the female, or the female named "female" without the male. For woman is man's work, and man is the solace of woman's eyes; and neither of them could exist without the other.[4]

The interesting point here is that the relationship between women and men is compared to the relationship between humankind and God. Granted, hierarchy defines both the relations between men and women and those between God and humankind,[5] since God (compared to human beings) and men (compared to women) are so strong that they can destroy the universe and other beings in irreversible ways, as indicated in Hildegard's interpretation of original sin; if Adam had sinned first, then humankind would not have had any hope, because of his stubbornness. God and men are like fire.

---

3 Hildegard of Bingen, *Causes and Cures*, trans. Throop, 68. "Nam cum deus soporem in Adam misit, anima eius in uera prophetia interim multa uidit, quia nondum aliquod peccatum habebat." Hildegard of Bingen, *Beate Hildegardis Cause et cure*, ed. Moulinier and Berndt, bk. 2, §164, p. 121. Hildegard of Bingen, *Causes and Cures*, trans. Throop, 111. "Cum enim Adam inspexit Euam, totus sapientia inpletus est, quia matrem, per quam filios procreare debebat, inspexit." Hildegard of Bingen, *Beate Hildegardis Cause et cure*, ed. Moulinier and Berndt, bk. 2, §164, p. 121.

4 Newman's translation, from Newman, *Sister of Wisdom*, 96. See Hildegard of Bingen, *Liber divinorum operum*, ed. Derolez and Dronke, pt. 1, bk. 4, chap. 100, p. 243: "Quia uir sine femina uir non uocaretur, nec femina sine uiro femina nominaretur. Femina enim opus uiri est, et uir aspectus consolationis femine est; et neuter eorum absque altero esse posset." Interestingly, this reciprocal relation is also applicable to God and his work, the human being, according to Hildegard's explanation of the relation between the body and the soul. "The soul by no means is without the body, just as God in no way is without work. He hid his work in himself before the ages and eternally in the ages. In the same way, the soul lies hidden, invisible in the body." Hildegard of Bingen, *Causes and Cures*, trans. Throop, 55. "Et sicut anima nullatenus sine corpore, sic et deus nullo modo sine opere est. Opus enim suum ante euum in euo eternaliter in ipso latuit, quemadmodum anima inuisibiliter in corpore latet." Hildegard of Bingen, *Beate Hildegardis Cause et cure*, ed. Moulinier and Berndt, bk. 2, §130, p. 101.

5 Hildegard attributes the creation to fire, and she compares God and men to fire. "He is that Fire from which every fire that provides for happiness is kindled, as sparks come forth from fire." Hildegard of Bingen, *Book of Divine Works*, trans. Campbell, 282. "Et ignis ille est, a quo omnis ignis qui ad beatitudinem respicit assenditur, quemadmodum scintillę ab igne procedunt." Hildegard of Bingen, *Liber divinorum operum*, ed. Derolez and Dronke, pt. 2, bk. 1, chap. 14, p. 281.

It is only women and humankind that can mitigate the destructive power of men and God. In the *Book of Divine Works*, Hildegard says, "fire burns with such force that it would spare nothing if it were not tempered by the water. And as water attends to fire by sparing, so too humanity was joined to divinity to be spared"[6] Of course, fire and water are both necessary. Fire gives humankind light and warmth, while water provides people with blood and flow. "Water manifests heat in a person's blood, air in his breathing, moisture in his perfected state, inundation in cleansing, quickness in vivification, sap in strengthening, predilection in bringing forth fruit, vital force in erection, moisture in strength, and dampness in all joints."[7]

Interestingly, men and God are similar in that they are fire. "For God, who is fire and light, vivifies the human person through the soul and moves him through rationality."[8] Men in Hildegard's *Cause et cure* have sexual desire like fire, which is stirred inside the man's body. The testicles attest to the heat, and the penis has fire, which can be overabundant or too violent.[9] "Delectation in a man is similar to fire, which sometimes is extinguished, sometimes flames up; constantly burning fire would consume many things."[10] On the other hand, women and humankind are strongly characterized by water, which is often represented as purgative. The Great Flood in Genesis

---

6 Hildegard of Bingen, *Book of Divine Works*, trans. Campbell, 284. "Et ignis in tanta ui ardet, ut nulli parceret nisi per aquam temperaretur. Et ut aqua igni parcendo adest, sic etiam humanitas diuinitati adiuncta est." Hildegard of Bingen, *Liber divinorum operum*, ed. Derolez and Dronke, pt. 2, bk. 1, chap. 15, p. 283.

7 Hildegard of Bingen, *Causes and Cures*, trans. Throop, 37. "Sic aqua in sanguine hominis calorem, in spiratione eius aerem, in perfectione humorem, in purgatione inundationem, in uegetatione uelocitatem, in confortatione succum, in fructificatione gustum, in erectione uiriditatem, in fortitudine humiditatem ac in omnibus compaginibus ipsius humectationem manifestat." Hildegard of Bingen, *Beate Hildegardis Cause et cure*, ed. Moulinier and Berndt, bk. 2, §82, p. 74.

8 Hildegard of Bingen, *Book of Divine Works*, trans. Campbell, 285. "Nam Deus ignis et lux existens per animam hominem uiuificat et per racionalitatem eum mouet." Hildegard of Bingen, *Liber divinorum operum*, ed. Derolez and Dronke, pt. 2, bk. 1, chap. 15, p. 283.

9 Hildegard explains that the testicles might have issues such as an ulcer or swelling if a man's sexual pleasure is excessive and causes dampness. Hildegard of Bingen, *Causes and Cures*, trans. Throop, 83; Hildegard of Bingen, *Beate Hildegardis Cause et cure*, ed. Moulinier and Berndt, bk. 2, §215, p. 140.

10 Hildegard of Bingen, *Causes and Cures*, trans. Throop, 59. "Nam delectatio in uiro igni assimulatur, qui interdum extinguitur; interdum ascenditur, qui ignis, qui assidue arderet, multa consumeret." Hildegard of Bingen, *Beate Hildegardis Cause et cure*, ed. Moulinier and Berndt, bk. 2, §143, p. 106.

was created to wipe out sinful creatures. "and it [creation] is sustained by the water that washes all things clean."[11] In particular, the female body is known for its strong moisture, while the male body is drier. And of course, women's menstruation, the peak of blood, is a purgative process, stressing women's watery nature.

Along the same lines, sexual desire and pleasure function differently according to sex and gender, and they have to be mutual. Hildegard sees the proper exchange of fluids and emotions as positive, and even necessary to health and reproduction. For Hildegard, sexual pleasure itself is not merely a necessary evil, as we saw above. Rather, Hildegard sees it as a necessary *good* for both men and women to have enough pleasure to emit semen or foam and conceive a child. Pleasure is important not just because it arouses but also because it affects the partners through their bodies. Without partners, sexual desire falls into nothing. There should be a consensus and mutual arousal between partners. If only one or the other enjoys sexual intercourse, or neither of them does, it does not provide the proper physical environment needed to produce healthy babies.[12]

According to *Cause et cure*, sexual pleasure is produced from the marrow; then, it travels around the body. The genitals of women and men receive it. However, the mechanism is slightly different in the two sexes. For men, lust is like a storm and fire, which are poured into the genitals.[13] On the other

11 Hildegard of Bingen, *Book of Divine Works*, trans. Campbell, 284. "Ipsique aqua adest, quę omnia mundat." Hildegard of Bingen, *Liber divinorum operum*, ed. Derolez and Dronke, pt. 2, bk. 1, chap. 15, p. 283.

12 As for many other medieval theologians, sexual desire and pleasure are only for having offspring for Hildegard. However, this does not mean that she saw them as evil, as many male theologians did. For her, they are needed for reproduction and therefore necessary. Unless they go beyond the norm, they are encouraged. However, she sees that not every person is the same in having pleasure or sexual desire. For instance, melancholic women are not suitable for intense sexual pleasure. "If these women at any time have delectation of the flesh, it quickly ceases." Hildegard of Bingen, *Causes and Cures*, trans. Throop, 73. "Et si iste ad horam aliquam delectationem carnis habuerint, cito tamen in eis deficit." Hildegard of Bingen, *Beate Hildegardis Cause et cure*, ed. Moulinier and Berndt, bk. 2, §175, p. 128.

13 "When the storm of lust rises in a male, it circles around in him like a mill. His loins are like a workshop in which marrow sends out fire. That workshop pours the fire into the genital regions of the male, and makes him burn ardently." Hildegard of Bingen, *Causes and Cures*, trans. Throop, 63. "Nam cum tempestas libidinis in masculo surgit, in eo ut molendinum circumuoluitur, quia etiam lumbi eius uelut fabrica sunt, in quam medulla ignem mittit, ita quod et fabrica illa eundum ignem in genitalia loca masculi transfundit ac eum fortiter ardere facit." Hildegard of Bingen, *Beate Hildegardis Cause et cure*, ed. Moulinier and Berndt, bk. 2, §151, p. 114.

hand, women's lust is gentler and similar to wind, which is not dissimilar to Eve's airy nature.[14] The female libido goes through a more complicated process because the womb into which it falls is "spacious" and resembles an "open space" (*apertum locum*) so that it can be expanded.[15] It is to receive the flow of semen and hold the fertilized egg.

Hildegard argues that women's lust is more flexible and adjustable to circumstances. First, women's lust is weaker for physical and societal reasons. Women's bodies are smaller; therefore, their bodily desires are smaller. And women's desire is easily controlled "either through fear or shame."[16] The physical needs of women are open to change more easily, according to their circumstances, and can result in a lack of ejaculation when there is no physical contact with men. Hildegard says, "Her wind is windy [volatile], her veins are open, and her body parts are more pliable than a man's," after asserting that "[t]he woman is only a vessel, so that she might conceive and give birth,"[17] emphasizing flow.

These sex and gender differences are applied to the different sex and gender roles attached to women and men, still emphasizing women's role as vessels. However, this vessel imagery does not represent women

---

14 It is interesting that Hildegard brings up the notion of a cloud, which is a mixture of water and air, to denote Eve's creation from Adam's body. An illustration in the Rutenberg codex of her *Scivias* shows a cloud with stars above when Eve was born out of Adam's side.

15 "But, when the wind of delectation leaves the marrow of a woman, it falls into the womb, where in adheres to the navel, and moves the woman's blood to carnal desire. Because the womb is spacious around the woman's navel, and has something like an open spot, the wind in her womb swells." Hildegard of Bingen, *Causes and Cures*, trans. Throop, 63–64. "Sed cum uentus delectationis ex medulla femine egreditur, in matricem, que umbilico adheret, cadit et sanguinem mulieris ad delectationem mouet, et quia matrix circa umbilicum mulieris amplum et uelut apertum locum habet, uentus ille in uentrem eius se dilatat." Hildegard of Bingen, *Beate Hildegardis Cause et cure*, ed. Moulinier and Berndt, bk. 2, §151, p. 114.

16 "She is able to hold herself back from delectation more easily than a man, either through fear or shame." Hildegard of Bingen, *Causes and Cures*, trans. Throop, 64. "Et ideo etiam aut pre timore aut pre pudore facilius quam uir a delectatione se continere ualet." Hildegard of Bingen, *Beate Hildegardis Cause et cure*, ed. Moulinier and Berndt, bk. 2, §151, p. 114.

17 "The woman is only a vessel, so that she might conceive and give birth. Her wind is volatile, her veins are open, and her body parts are more pliable than a man's." Hildegard of Bingen, *Causes and Cures*, trans. Throop, 64. "Quia femina tantum uas est, ut prolem concipiat et pariat, ac ideo etiam uentus eius uentosus est ut uene aperte atque membra eius solubiliora sunt quam uiri." Hildegard of Bingen, *Beate Hildegardis Cause et cure*, ed. Moulinier and Berndt, bk. 2, §151, p. 115.

as empty, passive entities, but as active in conceiving, moderating, and empowering God's words and new life.[18] Men's sexual and reproductive roles are like summer, to effuse and fructify, just as because Adam was made of earth, so he produces from earth. Their sexual acts are circular, flowing constantly through each other in the same way that "[t]he air is moved by the wind, and the wind is mingled with the air, so that in their movement all verdant things are subject to their influence."[19] Woman was created from the body of man, and men are born from women's wombs.[20] On the other hand, women's equivalent role resembles what winter does; women keep and save the elements produced by earth and men.[21] While women's and men's roles are reciprocal, the female body functions more like a container. This container is physical because through it women bear

18 For more on the activeness of the vessel image in Hildegard of Bingen's writings, see Minji Lee, "The Womb in Labour," 1183–99.

19 Hildegard of Bingen, *Scivias*, trans. Hart and Bishop, 78. "Aer de uento mouetur, et uentus aeri implicatur, ita quod in ambitu eorum quaeque uiridia illis subdita sunt." Hildegard of Bingen, *Scivias*, ed. Führkötter and Carelvaris, pt. 1, bk. 2, chap. 12, p. 21.

20 Whether Hildegard intended to or not, she emphasizes the complementary positions of women and men by misquoting 1 Corinthians 11:8–9. According to Newman, while Paul states that "man was not made from woman, but woman from man. Neither was man created for man, but woman for man," Hildegard states instead in her exegesis: "As the woman is of the man, so is the man for the woman; but all are from God (I Cor. 11:12)." In this part, Hildegard suggests that both women and men are made for each other. She presents reproduction as the most profound example of this mutual partnership: "The wife must cooperate with the husband and the husband with the wife in making children." Then she follows up with the sinful act of infidelity. Hildegard of Bingen, *Scivias*, trans. Hart and Bishop, 78. "*Sicut mulier de uiro ita et uir per mulierem, omnia autem ex Deo*....Mulier uiro et uir mulieri in opere filiorum cooperatur." Hildegard of Bingen, *Scivias*, ed. Führkötter and Carelvaris, pt. 1, bk. 2, chap. 12, p. 21. Newman also explained the woman's and man's complementary roles in the Hildegardian understanding of reproduction. Newman, *Sister of Wisdom*, 94–99.

21 "For through winter and summer fruits grow and are brought forth, and without them no fruit could mature. It is also through the tree's root, which keeps viridity within itself, that flowers and fruits are nurtured, and they are from a single source. So are many produced by male and female, yet they come forth from a single Creator." Hildegard of Bingen, *Book of Divine Works*, trans. Campbell, 332–33. "Per hiemem enim et estatem fructus crescunt et proferuntur, et absque istis nulli perficiuntur. Per radicem quoque arboris, quę uiriditatem in se continet, flores et poma enutriuntur, et ab uno sunt; ita per masculum et feminam multi procreantur, qui tamen ab uno creatore procedunt." Hildegard of Bingen, *Liber divinorum operum*, ed. Derolez and Dronke, pt. 2, bk. 1, chap. 43, p. 329.

offspring. At the same time, this container is spiritual in that women bear prophetic knowledge.[22]

According to Hildegard, reproduction is possible only when absorption and release happen properly through the parents' bodies, in particular the woman's body. During intercourse, the male partner has to send his semen to the female partner, while the female needs both actions—bringing in and sending out.[23] In medieval physiology, it was controversial whether women have semen or not. Hildegard did not believe in women's semen. Instead, she argues that women release a kind of foam when they are aroused during intercourse. Sexual pleasure itself is also the result of sexual desire coming out of the designated organ. In fact, sexual pleasure itself is the aftermath of original sin, when the first human beings swallowed the forbidden fruit and received sin and its harmful effects in their bodies. As a result, women must endure the reproductive process, eventually sending a baby out from their bodies into the world.

In the process of intercourse, the woman's and man's affections and sexual fluids flow into each other so that they can intermingle and become one flesh. The woman's blood draws and embraces the man's seed by the power of love, so that it can mix with the semen. At the same time, the male partner's body is warmed by the female partner's arousal and drawn to the woman's body, while his blood, "liquified, flows about and is turned around

---

22 "When Adam looked at Eve, he was completely filled with knowledge, because he looked at the mother through whom he should procreate children. When Eve looked at Adam, she looked into him, as if she looked into the sky and, since her hope was in the man, just as a soul, which desires heavenly things, tends upward." Hildegard of Bingen, *Causes and Cures*, trans. Throop, 111. "Cum enim Adam inspexit Euam, totus sapientia impletus est, quia matrem, per quam filios procreare debebat, inspexit. Cum autem Eua inspexit Adam, sic eum inspexit, quasi in celum uideret, et ut anima sursum tendit, que celestia desiderat, quoniam spes eius erat ad uirum." Hildegard of Bingen, *Beate Hildegardis Cause et cure*, ed. Moulinier and Berndt, bk. 2, §283, p. 176. It is also during Adam's initial sleep that he conceived Eve through a vision of prophetic knowledge, according to Hildegard. "Nam cum deus soporem in Adam misit, anima eius in uera prophetia interim multa uidit, quia nondum aliquod peccatum habebat. Ita et dormiente homine anima eius in uera prophetia multa uideret, si idem homo peccatis grauatus non esset." Hildegard of Bingen, *Beate Hildegardis Cause et cure*, ed. Moulinier and Berndt, bk. 2, §164, p. 121.

23 For this reason, Galenic physiology asserts that the female partner must have more pleasure than the male partner, as the woman performs two different actions, releasing and absorbing, while the man only ejaculates.

like a mill."[24] This process of attraction, liquification, and blending is necessary to make the partners' blood and body one, as the Scriptures describe: "For this cause shall a man leave his father and mother, and shall be joined unto his wife, and they two shall be one flesh" (Ephesians 5:31). And this one flesh will be embodied as a baby with one flesh.

> The fact that the man and woman have become, and are one flesh, was lying hidden in the man's side, from which the woman, taken, was made his flesh. The man and woman more easily flow together for conceiving in their blood and sweat. The power of eternity, which brings forth the infant from its mother's womb, makes the man and woman one flesh.[25]

Eve flowed out of Adam's body, becoming one body. A legitimate couple should become flexible and melt like water in terms of flesh and blood, which will enable them to flow into each other. Like Adam and Eve, if the partners are already one body, they can flow into each other more easily to become one flesh and one blood.[26] In this description, the flesh should be so softened and blood should be so flowing that both sexes can mingle with each other, when the images of softness and flow are much closer to the characterization of women. Eve and her female offspring have softer flesh than Adam and his offspring. Women also regularly experience the flow of blood during their fertile years: menstruation. Then, this softness and flow are required for two partners to become one blood and one body and produce children in Hildegard's view.

---

24 Hildegard of Bingen, *Causes and Cures*, trans. Throop, 57. "Sanguis eius liquefactus diffluit atque, ut molendinum circumuolutus." Hildegard of Bingen, *Beate Hildegardis Cause et cure*, ed. Moulinier and Berndt, bk. 2, §139, p. 104.

25 Hildegard of Bingen, *Causes and Cures*, trans. Throop, 57. "Quod autem uir et mulier una caro sic fiunt et sunt, hoc in latere uiri latitabat, ubi mulier de latere uiri sumpta caro eius facta est, ac ideo uir et mulier tanto facilius ad conceptionem in sanguine et sudore suo sic in unum confluent. Sed uis eternitatis, que infantem de uentre matris sue educit, uirum et feminam sic unam carnem facit." Hildegard of Bingen, *Beate Hildegardis Cause et cure*, ed. Moulinier and Berndt, bk. 2, §139, p. 104.

26 Hildegard insists that if either a woman or a man has coitus outside marriage, the resulting offspring is often unhappy, because the blood was drawn into the wrong partner. This psychological side effect in the children is caused by contamination and pollution that are compared to Adam and Eve's first sin. In general, Hildegard refers specifically to Adam in connection with the pollution arising from original sin, or sometimes Eve, but this time Adam and Eve are both mentioned to emphasize that this can happen to both men and women. Hildegard of Bingen, *Causes and Cures*, trans. Throop, 57–58. Hildegard of Bingen, *Beate Hildegardis Cause et cure*, ed. Moulinier and Berndt, bk. 2, §§139–41, pp. 104–5.

Women's Contribution in Re-creation

Hildegard does not think that women have semen like men, but there is nevertheless a feminine contribution to conception. For her, the woman's blood is too weak to produce seed. Instead, women make "a small thin foam."[27] However, she does not quite echo Aristotle and his followers, who thought that women simply provided the material for the embryo while men donated vitality and motion; it is clear that a woman's role matters in reproduction, affecting the outcome in various ways, even if Hildegard still accepts the popular image of sex as an agricultural process in which men are the farmers and women are the fields to be ploughed.[28] Even as women were traditionally regarded as having a simpler task, such as supplying materials to a baby or carrying a baby until delivery, Hildegard sees their contribution in various aspects, including their emotional state, making affection a condition of successful reproduction.

Even at the moment of conception, Hildegard relates the health of the baby both to the condition of the semen and to the affection of the partners. And she continues to focus on the importance of flow in this process as well. She describes the moment of conception in this way:

> When a man, approaching a woman for pouring forth his strong semen, has correct loving esteem for the woman, and the woman at the same time holds the man in loving esteem, a male is conceived, because it has been so ordained by God. It cannot be otherwise, since Adam was formed from mud, a stronger material than flesh. This male child will be prudent and virtuous, because he was conceived from strong semen and correct loving esteem of both parents.[29]

---

27 Hildegard of Bingen, *Causes and Cures*, trans. Throop, 51. "Sed de recta natura mulieris sanguis eius, quia debilis et tenuis est, semen non habet, sed tantum tenuem et paruam spumam emittit." Hildegard of Bingen, *Beate Hildegardis Cause et cure*, ed. Moulinier and Berndt, bk. 2, §129, p. 96.

28 Hildegard of Bingen, *Causes and Cures*, trans. Throop, 86. "Nam femina est nunc uelut terra aratro arata et semen uiri suscipit et in sanguinem suum inuoluit et calore suo calefacit, et sic illud crescit, dum spiraculum uite in ipsum mittitur et dum maturum tempus uenit, ut procedat." Hildegard of Bingen, *Beate Hildegardis Cause et cure*, ed. Moulinier and Berndt, bk. 2, §225, p. 144.

29 Hildegard of Bingen, *Causes and Cures*, trans. Throop, 30. "Nunc autem cum uir in effusione fortis seminis sui et in recto amore caritatis, quam ad mulierem habet, ad ipsam accedit, muliere quoque rectum amorem ad uirum tunc in eadem hora habente, masculus concipitur, quia sic a deo ordinatum est. Nec aliter fieri potest, quin masculus concipiatur, quoniam et Adam formatus est de limo, qui fortior materia est quam caro. Et hic masculus prudens et uirtuosus erit, quia sic in forti

She then continues to explain different cases according to these conditions. Whether the man's semen is strong or weak determines the sex of the baby. If the man's semen is strong, a male child is made; if the man's semen is weak, a female child is born. Likewise, the strength of the woman's love for the man during intercourse establishes the bodily condition of the child. Only if the woman truly loves her partner in coitus is a healthy child born. If the woman does not have strong affection and love for the man during coitus, the baby is weakened. A baby is born with a gender and character influenced by the different conditions of the parents.

> If, however, love for the man is lacking in the woman, so that only the man has the correct loving esteem for the woman at that time, and if the semen of the man is strong, a male is nevertheless conceived, because the loving esteem of the man is pre-eminent. But that male child will be weak and not virtuous, since love for the man was lacking in the woman. If the semen of the man is weak, even if he has the proper love for the woman, and she for him, a virtuous [strong] female is produced. If only one parent has the proper love for the other, and the semen of the male is weak at the time, a female is born because of the debility of the semen.[30]

It is interesting that Hildegard considers the feelings of the woman towards her husband as well as her physical condition as important factors in the character of the offspring. Whether or not the woman is fond of her partner is considered to be a critical aspect of the production of healthy children.

After noting that women do not have semen but a foamy fluid that is expelled when they are aroused during intercourse, Hildegard goes on to explain how women contribute to the formation of the embryo by providing a space for its development and nutrition until it develops into a baby. The

---

semine ac in recto amore caritatis utrorumque, quem ad inuicem habent, conceptus est." Hildegard of Bingen, *Beate Hildegardis Cause et cure*, ed. Moulinier and Berndt, bk. 2, §63, pp. 62–63.

30 Hildegard of Bingen, *Causes and Cures*, trans. Throop, 30. "Si autem hic amor deest in muliere ad uirum, ita quod tantum uir rectum amorem caritatis in ipsa hora ad mulierem habet et non mulier ad uirum, et si semen uiri forte est: masculus tamen concipitur, quia amor caritatis uiri superexcellit, sed idem masculus debilis erit et non uirtuosus, quoniam hic amor in muliere ad uirum defuit. Quoniam si semen uiri tenue est, qui tamen amorem caritatis ad illum, ibi femina uirtuosa procreatur. Si uero amor caritatis uiri est ad mulierem et non mulieris ad uirum, uel si amor caritatis in muliere est ad uirum et non uiri ad mulierem, semen autem uiri in ipsa hora tenue; item femina ex hoc nascitur propter debilitatem seminis." Hildegard of Bingen, *Beate Hildegardis Cause et cure*, ed. Moulinier and Berndt, bk. 2, §63, p. 63.

uterus is not a motionless, functionless, empty room. Instead, a woman's body closely engages with the fertilized egg so that it can fully develop into a baby with new life. In this process, the four humours present in the woman's body (which originate from the four elements of the universe) surround the mixture of female foam and male semen, which will be more fully discussed later. The important aspect to note here is that Hildegard appreciates that the process takes place in women's reproductive bodies.

The mother's importance to the growing foetus is discussed by other medieval writers; however, the mother's function is often limited to contributing the matter from which the foetus is formed. Aristotle saw the mother's body only as a house for its storage and the father's semen as providing the generative power and form to the embryo, blaming the cold nature of the woman's body for its inability to produce a seed.[31] It might be easier to find appreciation of women's reproductive role in medieval texts than in ancient ones,[32] but medieval men still dismiss the life-giving part of women's contribution. For them, it was men who performed more essential work in giving life to a foetus. For example, Pseudo-Albertus Magnus seems to neglect the mother's role when he talks about the three stages of the embryo's development.[33] By contrast, Hildegard provides readers with detailed descriptions of what occurs during pregnancy, emphasizing the close connections between the mother and foetus. Hildegard argues that the womb is the place that provides the egg, foetus, and baby with physical modification, spiritual preparation, and God's power of eternity, and although Hildegard emphasizes the non-material functions of the woman's body in reproduction, she also acknowledges the importance of the womb as a provider of material contributions such as nutrition.

---

31 York, *Health and Wellness*, 62.

32 Vaughan, *Women, Food, and Diet*, 51.

33 A famous medieval physician who was active slightly later than Hildegard, Pseudo-Albertus Magnus stated that in the first stage the embryo develops with "the vegetative power of the soul, and this vegetative power is derived from the father or from the one who engendered by means of sperm," referring to Aristotle's *On the Soul*. In the second and third stages, the embryo acquires a sensitive power from its soul and an intellective power from heaven, but the author still does not mention any power originating from the mother. Instead, when he talks about the mother's role in the growing foetus, he focuses on the negative effects a mother may have, such as women who corrupt the embryo through menses, the arts of midwifery, evil deeds, and excessive sexual pleasure. See Pseudo-Albertus Magnus, *Women's Secrets*, trans. Lemay, 102–3. Pseudo-Albertus, *De secretis mulierum*, 83–85.

In her section on conception, Hildegard describes how when men's semen is intermingled with women's foam, semen's toxic properties are neutralized by women's foam and the four elements surrounding it, and as a result, it becomes an embryo and eventually a baby with bodily members and organs. Here, a woman's reproductive role is important in providing not only the place for development but also the foam, elemental composition, and nutrition for the embryo. Although Hildegard refers to a woman's body as a "vessel," it is not just that: it is an active entity that has a crucial role in developing the mixture of semen and foam and forming it into a substance that will become a fully formed baby.

> From the mother's heat the fetus, not yet alive, develops in the rich matter of coagulation, while staying in the already mentioned heat. This is the work of one month, namely the time during which the moon waxes and wanes. The coagulation grows and becomes fatty. If it were not animated in this rich matter, it would be totally dried up. From the mother's dryness it would become slow and sorrowful.[34]

Hildegard emphasizes the interactions between the mother and the embryo. The mother's condition is important in providing the necessary care.

First, the woman's body is responsible for detoxifying the poisonous nature of semen to generate new life. Contrary to the theologians and medical theorists of her time, Hildegard finds pollution in the man's body, not the woman's, as God's punishment. In medieval medicine and religion, it was commonly believed that women's menstrual blood was not only polluted but also polluting, a belief that originated in ancient Greco-Roman medicine. For example, Pliny the Elder lists the harmful effects that women can cause with their periods. Possible consequences of this "venom" in women's menstrual fluid include a predisposition for epilepsy and leprosy in children conceived during menstruation. When Pseudo-Albertus Magnus advises men not to have intercourse with women during their periods (after providing tips for recognizing whether a woman is menstruating or not), he offers the following cautionary information:

> And let any man watch out that he does not have sex then [at the time of menstruation], because children who are conceived during the menstrual

34 Hildegard of Bingen, *Causes and Cures*, trans. Throop, 52. "De calore enim matris in pinguedinem coagulationis proficit nondum uiuens, sed in prefato calore persistens, et hoc opus in uno mense est, scilicet quo luna crescit et deficit. Et sic etiam predicta coagulatio crescit et pinguescit, quoniam, si in hac pinguedine non uiuificaretur, tota siccaretur, de qua siccitate mater multum tarda et dolens efficeretur." Hildegard of Bingen, *Beate Hildegardis Cause et cure*, ed. Moulinier and Berndt, bk. 2, §129, p. 97.

> flow will have a greater tendency to epilepsy and leprosy. And these sorts of infirmities are inflicted more quickly than any other leprosy, for which reason due to the toxicity of such women it is harmful to go to bed with them.[35]

Commentary B supports Pseudo-Albertus Magnus's view in detail, explaining that menstrual substances are composed of pure and impure elements. While pure elements have no issue of pollution and can feed the foetus, impure menses are dangerous, as they are made from a certain superfluity and impurity caused by non-digestion of food. Menstruation occurs because of the woman's inferior body, which lacks dryness and, above all, heat. The menstrual fluids are excrement produced after the humours have gone through physical processes. As Pseudo-Albertus Magnus emphasizes in his popular book, which was circulated among men, menstrual blood is known for its power to cloud mirrors and kill plants, animals, and even young babies.

Hildegard argues quite the opposite, although she does not list all of the side effects that noxious semen might bring. She suggests that the first human transgression had a much greater impact on the male body, turning semen poisonous. Hildegard justifies this argument by reminding readers of God's creation. God creates Adam with four elements, including earth with its hard nature, while Eve is born out of Adam's flesh. Therefore, Adam ends up with the stronger body, which comes with hardness and stubbornness. Due to this virile obstinacy, Adam receives the full blow of the aftermath of original sin in his body. Just as Eve's daughters inherit God's punishment of menstruation, Adam's sons inherit the punishment of polluted semen: "[p]artaking of evil, the blood of the sons of Adam transformed into poisonous semen, from which the sons of men are procreated."[36]

In order to create new life from this polluted semen, Hildegard suggests that detoxification is needed. For her, reproduction is repeated creation. Recalling the pure state of the first human beings, the fertilized egg should be

35 My translation of "Et caveat sibi quivis quod tunc non coeat, quia pueri qui in menstruis fluentibus concipiuntur maiorem inclinacionem habent ad morbum caducum et ad lepram. Et tales huiusmodi infirmitates qua alia cicius inficiuntur lepra, quare propter talem venenositatem mulierum nocivum est coire." Pseudo-Albertus Magnus, *El "De secretis mulierum,"* trans. Barragán Nieto, chap. 8, §§27–28, p. 448n.

36 Hildegard of Bingen, *Causes and Cures*, trans. Throop, 31. "Nam de gustu mali uersus est sanguis filiorum Ade in uenenum seminis, de quo filii hominum procreantur." Hildegard of Bingen, *Beate Hildegardis Cause et cure*, ed. Moulinier and Berndt, bk. 2, §64, p. 64.

pure to receive a soul and fully develop. This essential process happens in the womb, immediately after intercourse when the semen falls into the woman's body. Here, the woman's heat cures the man's problem, inherited from Adam.

> These [uprisen humours] all create a tempest, from their excessive superfluity. From the blood, they bring forth a poisonous foam, which is semen. When it falls upon its place, the blood of the mother joins with it, from which it will be bloody.[37] The same degeneration did not happen to Eve because her flesh was not strong enough. In Adam's transgression, the strength in the male's genital member changed into a poisonous foam, and the female's blood changed to a *contrary* effusion. Because man's flesh was made from earth, his blood has semen of a strong and correct nature. A woman's blood is also of a correct nature.[38]

While both Adam and Eve once had a correct nature, Adam was the one whose reproductive power became degraded, due to his strong semen. Eve could avoid this degradation because she did not have semen, but instead, she ended up with menstrual and reproductive flows.

In the following paragraph, Hildegard provides additional explanation. Semen's poisonous nature originated when Adam committed the first sin. Semen is produced from the blood when it is stirred by pleasure, which originates from the forbidden fruit offered by the serpent. According to Hildegard, the disturbed blood sends out a "cold foam,"[39] which contains pol-

---

37 Hildegard of Bingen, *Causes and Cures*, trans. Throop, 51. "Et hec omnia de nimietate superfluitatis quasi tempestatem faciunt et de sanguine uenenosam spumam, quod semen est, educunt, quod, cum in locum suum cadit, sanguis mulieris illi se conuingit, et hoc sanguine erit." Hildegard of Bingen, *Beate Hildegardis Cause et cure*, ed. Moulinier and Berndt, bk. 2, §129, p. 95.

38 Modified from Hildegard of Bingen, *Causes and Cures*, trans. Throop, 51. Modification is in italics; Throop translated "contrarium" as "dangerous," which is not incorrect but which could be misunderstood as suggesting that the woman's menstrual flow is dangerous to others. Unlike many medieval elites, Hildegard does not emphasize the poisonous nature of menstruation, although she refers to many cases in which women's health is endangered by medical issues related to menstruation. So here, "contrary" is more "dangerous" to women, which can be translated as "hurtful, injurious" to women themselves. Hildegard uses "contrary" as the opposite of "correct, right," still implying degeneration and the aftermath of original sin. "Nam in transgressione Ade fortitudo uiri in genitali membro uersus est in uenenosam spumam, atque mulieris sanguis uersus est in contrariam effusionem. De forti enim et de recta natura uiri sanguis eius semen habet, quia de terra caro factus est. Sed de recta natura mulieris sanguis eius." Hildegard of Bingen, *Beate Hildegardis Cause et cure*, ed. Moulinier and Berndt, bk. 2, §129, pp. 95–96.

39 Hildegard of Bingen, *Causes and Cures*, trans. Throop, 51. Hildegard of Bingen, *Beate Hildegardis Cause et cure*, ed. Moulinier and Berndt, bk. 2, §129, p. 95.

lution. Fortunately, however, this cold is mitigated by the female partner's heat, which is relatively secure from the degenerate nature that the male partner gives to the egg. Moreover, it is not just the woman's heat that helps conception. The four elements and the humours in the woman's body are all engaged with the semen. After warming the semen and making it bloody, the woman's heat (derived from fire) warms the fertilized egg, while her breath (derived from air) dries it. Her liquid (derived from water) sends pure moisture to the egg, and her membrane (derived from earth) constrains it.[40] This process represents the important role played by the various aspects of the female body in conception.

As many ancient and premodern theorists assumed, Hildegard also believes that menstrual blood provides the necessary nutrients to the foetus. The menstrual substances are commonly described as food for the foetus, which also explains why menstruation does not occur during pregnancy. Interestingly, however, Hildegard describes this process as mediated by flow. The pregnant woman's blood is drawn all the way to her breasts and turns into milk, supplied by what she eats and drinks.[41] The woman's body is described as the vessel itself, through which different fluids and ingredients travel vertically.

Hildegard also notes that the womb is the place where the soul enters into the embryo so that it can grow as a human being. The soul does not accompany men's semen. It is the second month when the soul, the "breath of life," contacts the fertilized egg in the womb. The soul's work is fundamental at this point, because the soul divides the egg so it can progress into a more developed form. Therefore, this description implies that the man's semen was not entirely equipped with all of the required elements:

> Then, as God wills and has arranged to happen, comes the breath of life and, without the mother's knowledge, it touches that form, as a strong, warm

40 "It is as if a poisonous foam until fire, that is heat, warms it; and until air, that is breath, dries it; and until water, that is liquid, allows pure dampness to enter; and until the earth, that is a membrane, constrains it. And then it will be bloody—not totally blood, but combined with a bit of blood." Hildegard of Bingen, *Causes and Cures*, trans. Throop, 51. "Et tam diu quasi uenenosa spuma est, usque dum ignis, uidelicet calor, illud calefacit, et dum aer, uidelicet spiramen, illud exsiccat, et dum aqua, scilicet fluor, illi puram humiditatem admittit, et usque dum terra, scilicet cutecula, illud constringit. Et tunc sic erit sanguineum, id est non totum sanguis, sed aliquantulum sanguine permixtum." Hildegard of Bingen, *Beate Hildegardis Cause et cure*, ed. Moulinier and Berndt, bk. 2, §129, p. 96.

41 The same logic was applied to nursing women, as Hildegard also suggests that menstrual blood is used to produce mother's milk.

> wind; just as a wind noisily blowing against a wall. It pours itself in and dashes against all the joints of its limbs. The separate parts gently divide from each other; just as flowers divide themselves in the heat of the sun. There is still great weakness in this form. It cannot be moved, but lies, so it might sleep, and breathes slightly.[42]

After this section, Hildegard gives readers a more detailed description of how the embryo grows each month once the soul enters it. According to her, even after the embryo receives the soul, it cannot survive alone, since it is rather a formless lump. Therefore, the embryo continues to have a close connection with the mother until it fully develops and is released from her womb:

> Because the soul is sent into the body, it is breath. Sent by God, it receives merit through physical works, whether good or bad. These works are like a framework of merits. Just as, at first, a child does not know what *they* understand; when *they* are more mature, *they* receive intellect, which understands all things. And just as *they* embrace their works, examining and kissing them, and later are fatigued by old age; so the soul, advancing toward a more perfect state, goes forward. It is encircled by good deeds, as if by a royal cloak, and obscured by bad deeds, in the same way the earth is suffused with waters; and the same way waters flow in certain places, so the soul suffuses and excels the baby. The soul often sees future events through prophecy, when the outer eyes are closed, since it remembers it lives without the body.[43]

---

42 Hildegard of Bingen, *Causes and Cures*, trans. Throop, 52. "Deinde sicut deus uult et sicut fieri disposuit, uenit spiraculum uite et formam illam matre nesciente tangit ut uehemens calidus uentus, uelut uentus, qui in parietem cum sono flat ac se infundit et infligit in omnes compages membrorum forme illius. Et sic omnes diuisiones membrorum eiusdem forme a se suauiter ita diuiduntur, ut flores ad calorem solis se diuidunt. Sed et adhuc tanta imbecillitas in eadem forma est, quod moueri non potest, sed iacet, ut dormiat, et modice spirat." Hildegard of Bingen, *Beate Hildegardis Cause et cure*, ed. Moulinier and Berndt, bk. 2, §130, p. 97.

43 Modified from Hildegard of Bingen, *Causes and Cures*, trans. Throop, 38. "Cum enim anima in corpus mittitur, spiramen est, et a deo missum est, ac per corporalia opera, siue bona siue mala sunt, meritum accipit. Et hec opera quasi compago meritorum sunt. Sicut enim infans primo nescit, quod postea intelligit, quia, cum maturior erit, intellectum, qui omnia intelligit, capit, et sicut tunc opera sua considerando et osculando amplectitur et sicut postea de senectute fatigatur: sic anima per opera proficiendo procedit. Et de bonis operibus uelut regali amictu circumdatur, de malis uero obfuscatur, quemadmodum etiam terra aquis perfunditur; et quemadmodum aque in quibusdam locis fluunt, ita anima corpus perfundit et ipsum corpus excellit, sed et ipsa oculis exterioribus clausis cum prophetia multotiens future uidet, quia sine corpore se uiuere recordatur." Hildegard of Bingen, *Beate Hildegardis Cause et cure*, ed. Moulinier and Berndt, bk. 2, §87, p. 76.

This section may remind readers of God's creation story: God sent his breath into Adam to vivify his creature. In *Cause et cure*, the soul is often identified with breath in this way. This is just one instance of how Hildegard views women's re-creation process (not just conception but also childbirth) in relation to God's creation. In particular, the moment of childbirth resembles the moment when God created Eve from Adam's body:

> With childbirth imminent, the vessel in which the infant had been enclosed, is split. The power of eternity, which brought forth Eve from Adam's side, arriving soon, is present and overturns every corner of the dwelling place of the woman's body. All the joints of the woman's body become involved with that force and they assist it and open themselves. They hold themselves while the infant emerges, and then resume their former arrangement. While the infant emerges, his soul feels the power of eternity, and is happy.[44]

Hildegard emphasizes that it is the "power of eternity" which opens and closes the mother's whole body. This power not only releases the baby but also restores the compactness of the woman's joints after birth. Additionally, this power is felt by the newborn and makes the infant happy. It is the same power that God used to create Eve from Adam's body. This scene was the prototype of the birth that happens to every human being. However, once the power of eternity enters Eve's body, it is passed on to her female offspring. Here, Hildegard suggests that women are conduits of God's eternal creative power through the birthing process.

Woman's Life-Giving Body

Hildegard's descriptions of conception, pregnancy, and childbirth thus present the idea that a woman's body is active in receiving life-giving substances: semen and the soul. This active role should also be understood in relation to her concept of *viriditas*, which represents regenerative and salvational qualities embodying the moisture, flow, and fecundity essential for conception and growth. While this concept was adapted by other theolo-

44 Hildegard of Bingen, *Causes and Cures*, trans. Throop, 56. "Sed cum iam partus instat, uas, in quo infans clausus est, scinditur, et uis eternitatis, que Euam de latere Ade eduxit, mox ueniens adest atque omnes angulos habitaculi corporis mulieris de locis suis euertit. Et omnes compagines corporis mulieris fortitudini illi occurrunt et eam suscipiunt ac se aperiunt. Atque ita se continent, dum infans egrediatur, ac deinde iterum replicant se, ut prius fuerunt. Sed et anima infantis, interim dum infans egreditur, sentit uim eternitatis, que eam misit, ac interim leta est." Hildegard of Bingen, *Beate Hildegardis Cause et cure*, ed. Moulinier and Berndt, bk. 2, §134, p. 102.

gians before Hildegard, it is so central and widely accepted in Hildegard's theology and medical treatises that it becomes an overarching category for regenerative and salvational qualities.[45] She viewed *viriditas* as a regenerative and salvational quality, embodying the moisture, flow, and fecundity essential for conception and growth.[46] This contrasted with the male-centred gynaecological explanations of her time, which often reduced women's role to a mere container.

For Hildegard, *viriditas* often appears in opposition to *ariditas*, "dryness" or "being withered."[47] Like the medical theorists who preceded her and those of her own day, Hildegard also related moisture and humidity to women and dryness to men. This moisture, along with the flow of blood, which I regard as a highly characteristic feature of women in her view, was a guarantee of female fecundity.

Here, I argue that man's poisonous nature and woman's therapeutic role work together to make reproduction possible. Although Françoise Charmaille insists in her analysis of intersex in *Cause et cure* that the engendering power of *viriditas* is more closely attached to men,[48] I see the opposite in

45 *Viriditas* is related to the colour green and was used to refer to the greenness of healthy plants. Moulinier lists the famous premodern authors from classical antiquity onwards in whose writings *viriditas* appears. For further information, see Moulinier and Berndt, "Introduction," xi–cxiii, especially lxxxv. McAvoy and Newman argue that even before the concept of *viriditas*, there were some views, including in the writings of Bernard Silvestris of Tours (d. ca. 1148), according to which woman's power brought ideas into reality as material entities. McAvoy, *The Enclosed Garden*, 154; Newman, *God and the Goddesses*, 64.

46 McAvoy, *The Enclosed Garden*, 154.

47 Hildegard of Bingen, *Causes and Cures*, trans. Throop, 11. "Et ita cum eo incedunt usque ad signum libre, ubi uiriditas et ariditas quasi in libra sunt, ita quod uiriditas absedit et ariditas accedit." Hildegard of Bingen, *Beate Hildegardis Cause et cure*, ed. Moulinier and Berndt, bk. 1, §31, p. 36.

48 Charmaille, "Intersex between Sex and Gender." In this article, Charmaille argues that *viriditas* is related to the earth; therefore, it is more about Adam, whose nature originated from the earth. Charmaille explains *viriditas* as a "manly vigor," but I argue that this *viriditas* is only possible when heat from men and moisture from women are combined with each other. Charmaille interprets the concept of *viriditas* as the combination of greenness and vigour. For her, vigour and its adjective form "vigorous" are related to virility and to man's earthly nature as well as to the phlegmatic temperament. While I agree with Charmaille that Hildegard's notion of gender is rich and related to phlegm, I argue that *viriditas* is closely related to woman's reproductive power. On the other hand, there is a place in Hildegard's homilies where *viriditas* appears in association with "virile vigour" to emphasize God's great power of generation, in the homily on Luke 14:16–24 for the Third Sunday after

Hildegard of Bingen's gynaecology. I agree with Charmaille that the concept of *viriditas* is related to greenness and vigorousness,[49] but I do not see it as necessarily limited to *virtus*, the manly quality. Hildegard's interpretation of *viriditas* is closely tied to women's reproductive power and the Virgin Mary, rather than solely associated with men or virility. For Hildegard, *viriditas* was closely associated with the feminine power that nurtures babies in women's bodies.[50] This power extends to the Virgin Mary and is directly linked to the motherly Ecclesia that contains and saves sinful souls in Hildegard's visions. Moreover, Hildegard introduced herself as "*materna viriditas*."[51]

Pentecost, where Jesus uses the analogy of a great man hosting a banquet. However, this manly expression, "virile vigour," seems to be used to emphasize God's ability in every aspect, and the image of a woman's womb is also mentioned in the same passage: "Adam 'said' to creation: 'Go *out* in servitude into every circle and ambit of human deeds and into the bending of plants. Bind the earth fast so that it opens itself and may sprout everywhere with greenness [*viriditas*] and fruit, and even with the vigor of the most vigorous sap, namely wine. For the vine is more a plant than a tree, and like a plant it is both planted in the earth and nourished, so that the womb of complete comprehension may be full, which I comprehend in the world.' . . . 'I assert to all creatures "that none" of the virile vigor that dwells with creatures will touch the world, with the sense of touch in a way such that creation would obey them as it has obeyed me and will bring them such easy fruit as it did for me.'" "39. The Third Sunday after Pentecost," in Hildegard of Bingen, *Homilies on the Gospels*, 158–61. While virtue was traditionally related to manly vigour, McAvoy rightly indicates that the role of Virtue in Hildegard's *Symphonia* and the *Ordo virtutum* were composed for and performed by nuns in the Rupertsberg monastery, which can be read to highlight these virginal women's important roles in re-creating Eden as "flowers flourishing within the 'nobilissima viriditas' of Christ." McAvoy, *The Enclosed Garden*, 162. "O noble verdure, which grows from the Sun of splendor! Your clear serenity shines in the Wheel of Godhead, Your greatness is past all earthly understanding, And Heaven's wonders surround you in their embrace." Hildegard of Bingen, *Scivias*, trans. Hart and Bishop, 528. "O nobilissima uiriditas quae radicas in sole et quae in candida serenitate luces in rota, quam nulla terrena excellentia comprehendit, tu circumdata es amplexibus diuinorum mysteriorum." Hildegard of Bingen, *Scivias*, ed. Führkötter and Carelvaris, pt. 3, bk. 13, chap. 7, p. 620.

49 Mark Bradley explains the colour green and the related terms *viridis* (adjective) and *virens* (noun) in relation to vigour. Bradley, *Colour and Meaning in Ancient Rome*, 7–9.

50 McAvoy, *The Enclosed Garden*, 160.

51 "Now therefore, look to the Fiery Giver who endows mankind with discernment. What person can pit his voice against that which thundered above the heavens and overcame the abyss, ornamenting it with the covering of maternal fruitfulness [*materna uiriditas*]?" "Hildegard to Bernard and Gregory, Cardinals" in Hildegard of Bingen, *Letters*, trans. Baird and Ehrman, no. 7, 1:40. "Nunc ergo aspicite in igneum datorem, qui infundit bonum intellectum hominibus. Sed et quis homo potest conari

While Charmaille see the airy as the opposite of vigour and considers both airiness and lack of vigour to be female characteristics, I suggest that air is not far from vigorous power. In explaining the moon's effects on crops, Hildegard categorizes winds according to the different powers they receive from the moon. On the one hand, there is the wind that dries up plants in winter; on the other hand, there is the wind that brings forth *viriditas*, the greening power of growing plants.[52] Air is essential in germination, which is also connected to the airy nature of women in reproduction.

> Air has four powers: emitting dew, stirring up all greenness [*viriditas*], moving the breeze with which it brings forth flowers, and spreading heat with which it makes all things ripen, in the same way air itself is spread through the four parts of the world.[53]

This fecundity of the air is also related to Hildegard's emphasis on the relation between air and soul. After mixing earth, fire, and water, God blew air into the human form to vivify it with the spirit. Therefore, air functions to give vigour to plants: "[a]ir is the breath which, in dew, pours forth moisture to budding things, so that they all turn green. Through its breeze, it brings forth flowers and, through its heat, strengthens all things for maturity."[54] Even in her description of air's fecundity, Hildegard highlights flow. Air should blow and flow to make things germinate. The air whose nature it is to dry up trees and plants is an obstacle to fecundity in the same way as women whose bodily conditions are desiccated.

---

contra vocem illam, quae tonuit, ascendens supra alas, et quae abyssum superavit, sonans per tegmen maternae viriditatis?" Hildegard of Bingen, "Epistola XXXIV," 520. McAvoy, *The Enclosed Garden*, 175.

52 "Hildegard of Bingen, *Causes and Cures*, trans. Throop, 14. "Luna autem in se excipit feditatem inutilitatis aurarum et calorem puri aeris, stabilitatem utilis aure, pericula tempestatum, fortem aerem, qui omnnem uiriditatem profert, aerem, qui pomifera educit, aerem, qui exsiccat et defectum infert, qui hyemps est." Hildegard of Bingen, *Beate Hildegardis Cause et cure*, ed. Moulinier and Berndt, bk. 1, §37, p. 39.

53 Hildegard of Bingen, *Causes and Cures*, trans. Throop, 17. "Sed aer quatuor uires habet, uidelicet rorem emittendo, omnem uiriditatem excitando, flatum mouendo, cum quo flores educit, calorem dilatando, cum quo omnia maturescere facit; uelut et ipse per quatuor partes mundi dilatatur." Hildegard of Bingen, *Beate Hildegardis Cause et cure*, ed. Moulinier and Berndt, bk. 1, §43, pp. 43–44.

54 Hildegard of Bingen, *Causes and Cures*, trans. Throop, 17. "Aer enim spiramen est, quod in rore humorem germinantibus infundit, ita ut omnia uirescant, et quod per flatum flores educit et per calorem omnnia ad maturitatem confirmat." Hildegard of Bingen, *Beate Hildegardis Cause et cure*, ed. Moulinier and Berndt, bk. 1, §43, p. 44.

Just as the Hildegardian understanding of physical flow is closely connected to its salvational role, her concept of *viriditas* extends to the spirit, which is again related to air. Beverly Mayne Kienzle examined Hildegard's references to *viriditas*, which Kienzle translates as "the life-giving and animating force of greenness," in the *Homilies*.

> A taste of this richness can be savored in a brief summary of how the Homilies on the Gospels portray the Holy Spirit. The Spirit's circular motion guides all of salvation history with its life-giving power (Hom. 34). It directs the creation, moving with God across the waters (Hom. 34), tracing circles like the flight patterns of birds (Hom. 1), moving into the fastenings of the human body (Hom. 23) and whirling in the tempests of the soul within (Hom. 56), and, in several homilies, sending the virtues to rescue the sinful soul. The Spirit's light works miracles (Hom. 9), the small as well as the major events of salvation history. It animates the power of greenness in the universe, touching and kissing the sinful soul in need of healing (Hom. 19). Hence the Spirit participates in the work of creation and redemption. It also directs the transformation of history, which Hildegard saw as the transformation of the Scriptures from the Old Law to the New, accompanied by their interpretation according to spiritual understanding (Hom. 47).[55]

As seen in this concise overview of *viriditas* in Hildegard's teachings, this green power is deployed by the Holy Spirit to stimulate movement and regeneration in the bodies and souls of creatures. For Hildegard, *viriditas* is both renaturing and salvational, which I consider the power of the woman's reproductive body.

Hildegard's medical descriptions of conception and pregnancy provide the foundation for her theological claim that women are active, transformative participants in divine creation. Where male medical authorities emphasized women's passivity, Hildegard's careful attention to the womb's purifying and nurturing capacities reveals how physical processes embody broader spiritual truths. This medical–theological synthesis is central to her unconventional understanding and representation of women's bodies.

55 Kienzle, "Introduction," 7.

Chapter 5

GIVING BIRTH TO A BABY AND GIVING SPIRITUAL BIRTH TO HUMANKIND

IN *SCIVIAS*, HILDEGARD adapts the operations of a woman's body to represent the work of Ecclesia. Furthermore, the woman's reproductive role and its physical characteristics are used allegorically to explain the salvational function of Ecclesia. Hildegard's exegesis is somewhat novel insofar as it depicts women's reproductive processes more vividly than other theologians do, although she still relies on the traditional image of Ecclesia as a female figure. In medieval writing it is not difficult to find certain abstract Christian concepts or symbols, such as the Synagogue or Sophia, described as female characters.[1] Hildegard, however, adds a new dimension to this tradition by carefully exploring the allegorical potential of women's reproductive systems, providing her with new images showing how holiness may be contained in women's physical bodies. *Scivias*, specifically in the second book where Hildegard's vision depicts the present condition of human beings, shows in detail how Hildegard works with and changes standard conceptions of the woman's body as a vessel. In this vision, Hildegard describes Ecclesia as a female body and Ecclesia's salvational role as a distinctly feminine process of re-creation.

In her major vision in *Scivias*, Hildegard represents Ecclesia as having a woman's body going through purgation, pregnancy, and childbirth comparable to its salvational process. This vision highlights the medical notion of female porosity and religious ideas of female vulnerability, turning them into possibilities of redemption. Also, this femaleness in salvation is linked to Hildegard's understanding of God as a motherly figure, feeding people with milk. The holy representation of the female body, including the Virgin Mary's body, manifests the tension between porosity and integrity. While the virginal body of Jesus's mother had to be sealed, the possibility of pregnancy

1 In the first book of *Scivias*, Hildegard represents Synagogue as a pale blind woman. Although Synagogue is an important figure as "the mother of the Incarnation of the Son of God," Hildegard still uses her disability to identify her as "the holy forerunner" of the more important figure Ecclesia, following the medieval tradition of the Song of Songs. Hildegard of Bingen, *Scivias*, trans. Hart and Bishop, 133. "Quae est synagogal mater incarnationis Filii Dei" Hildegard of Bingen, *Scivias*, ed. Führkötter and Carelvaris, bk. 1, chap. 5, p. 94; Matter, *The Voice of My Beloved*, 92.

and childbirth in the lives of all women is seen by Hildegard as enabling the flows needed for health, salvation, and the celestial order by keeping the right balances and allowing motion to continue. In other words, the weaker female body allows flows so that it can conceive and be purged not just in physiological processes but also in cosmological and salvational ones.

The Salvational Flow of Ecclesia

Following medieval theological tradition, Hildegard represents Ecclesia in *Scivias* as female and identifies her with the Virgin Mary, as we have seen in the commentary tradition of the Song of Songs. However, what is unique about Hildegard's version of Ecclesia is her particularly vivid description of childbirth. While others may represent Ecclesia as female and compare Ecclesia's pain to labour, Hildegard's representation includes an unusual amount of detail and—even as an inversion of a normal process—shows she is thinking like a person with gynaecological knowledge. For her, the womb offers an important space to enable purification and to give people new life, in other words, salvation. Hildegard not only uses the traditional praises of the womb drawn from the Song of Songs but also develops this conventional and salvational idea into a more vividly physical representation.

Hildegard's description of Ecclesia characterizes her at once as a building, a queen, and a strangely perforated body. In this passage, the woman's body is not only positive but also redemptive. Here is Hildegard's description:

> After this I saw the image of a woman as large as a great city, with a wonderful crown on her head and arms from which a splendor hung like sleeves, shining from Heaven to earth. Her womb was pierced like a net with many openings, with a huge multitude of people running in and out. She had no legs or feet, but stood balanced on her womb in front of the altar that stands before the eyes of God, embracing it with her outstretched hands and gazing sharply with her eyes throughout all of Heaven.[2]

---

2 Hildegard of Bingen, *Scivias*, trans. Hart and Bishop, 169. "POST HAEC uidi quasi muliebrem imaginem tantae magnitudinis ut magna ciuitas est, habentem caput miro ornatu coronatum, et brachia de quibus splendor uelut manicae pendebat, a caelo usque ad terram radians. Venter autem eius erat in modum retis perforatus multis foraminibus, in quibus maxima multitudo hominum discurrebat. Crura uero et pedes non habebat, sed tantum super uentrem suum ante altare quod est ante oculos Dei stans, ipsum expansis manibus circumplectebatur, et oculis suis per omne caelum acutissime uidebat." Hildegard of Bingen, *Scivias*, ed. Führkötter and Carelvaris, pt. 2, bk. 3, p. 134.

But this is not a normal figure of a virgin queen:

> And that image spreads out its splendor like a garment, saying, "I must conceive and give birth!"
>
> Then I saw black children moving in the air near the ground like fishes in water, and they entered the womb of the image through the openings that pierced it. But she groaned, drawing them upward to her head, and they went out by her mouth, while she remained untouched. And behold, that serene light with her figure of a man in it, blazing with a glowing fire, which I had seen in my previous vision, again appeared to me, and stripped the black skin off each of them and threw it away; and it clothed each of them in a pure white garment and opened to them the serene light.[3]

Here, Hildegard reports that she saw Ecclesia as a womanly figure whose womb has many openings just like a net. In the same way that conception occurs (i.e., via uptake into the lower parts), in this passage Ecclesia draws sinful souls into her belly, or her womb, through its openings. When the souls pass through her body, they are cleansed and finally sent onwards to heaven through Ecclesia's mouth. These processes strongly evoke an image of childbirth; however, they are an alternative vision of it. We might also call this scene an inversion of the Virgin Mary's childbirth, perhaps relating to certain medieval beliefs that before delivering Jesus from her womb, Mary conceived through her mouth.[4]

While the womb is traditionally seen as a space of physiological vulnerability or danger, Hildegard inverts this view. The same permeability that once symbolized Eve's weakness now enables Ecclesia's redemptive labour. Through the act of receiving and transforming, the womb becomes a theological site of sanctification. And though Hildegard underscores Ecclesia's intact virginity—aligning her with the Virgin Mary—this does not contradict her openness. Instead, it reinforces the paradox at the heart of Hildegard's

---

3 Hildegard of Bingen, *Scivias*, trans. Hart and Bishop, 169. "Et eadem imago expandit splendorem suum uelut uestimentum dicens: 'Me oportet concipere et parere.'... Deinde uidi nigros infantes iuxta terram in aere quasi pisces in aqua pergentes, et uentrem eiusdem imaginis in foraminibus ubi perforata erat intrantes. At illa ingemuit, sursum eos ad caput suum trahens, ubi ad os eius exierunt, ipsa tamen integra permanente. Et ecce illa serena lux et in ipsa species hominis tota rutilante igne flagrans (secundum uisionem quam prius uideram) iterum mihi apparuit, et singulis eorum nigerrimam cutem abstrahens ac extra uiam easdem cutes proiciens, singulos illorum candidissima ueste induit ac eis serenissimam lucem aperuit." Hildegard of Bingen, *Scivias*, ed. Führkötter and Carelvaris, pt. 2, bk. 3, p. 135.

4 Constas, *Proclus of Constantinople and the Cult of the Virgin*, 278.

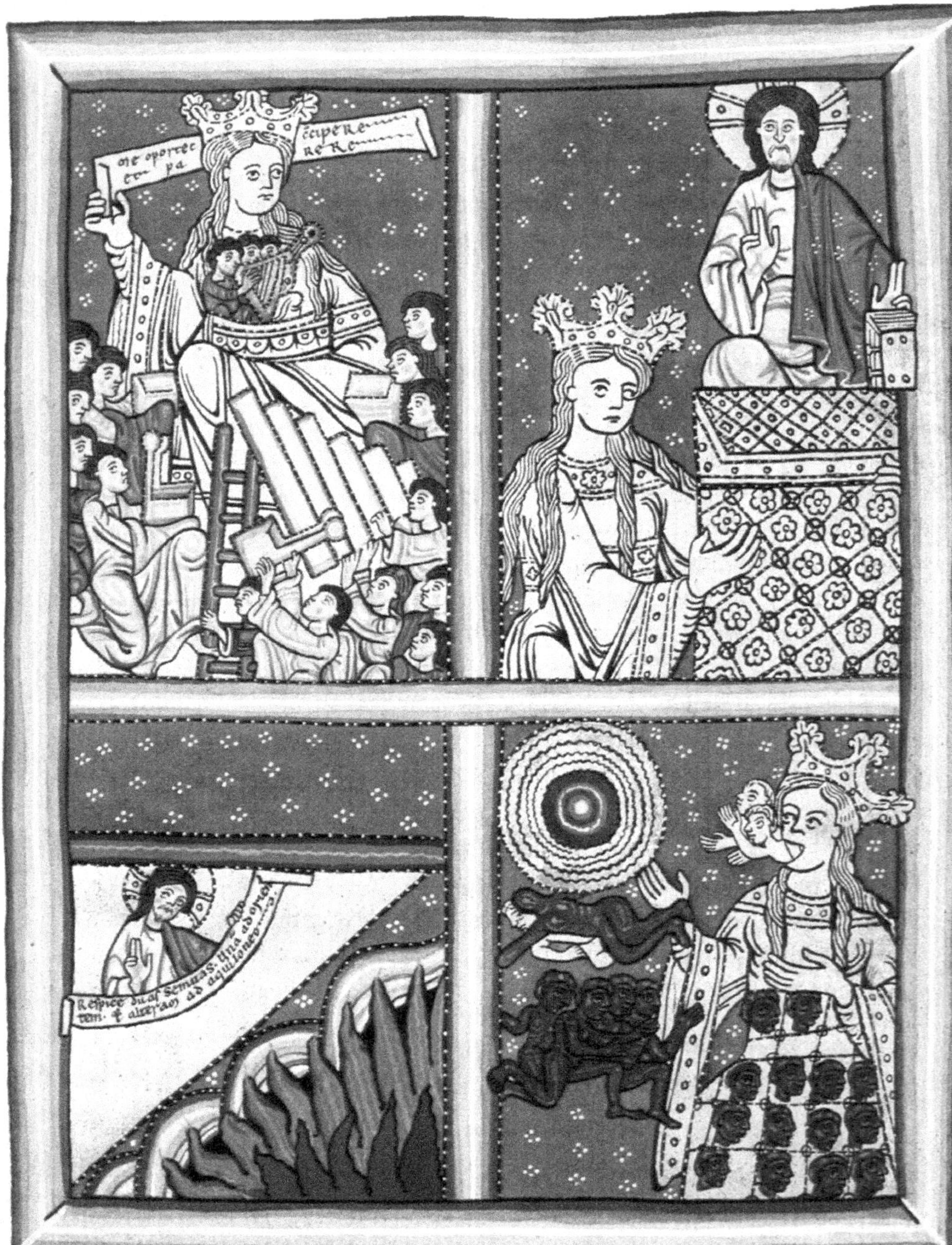

Figure 3. "Ecclesia, the Mother of the Faithful and Baptism."
In Hildegard of Bingen, *Scivias Codex*, pt. 2, vision 3, fol. 51r,
ca. 1175. Original lost, hand-copied on parchment, ca. 1930.
Rüdesheim-Eibingen, St. Hildegard's Abbey.
Courtesy of St. Hildegard's Abbey.

vision: a sealed virgin who is simultaneously a conduit, an ever-flowing vessel of divine grace.

Compared to actual bodily childbirth, this process in Hildegard's vision can be seen as soul rebirth. The difference is that this salvational process is done in the reverse order from physical childbirth. Still, the processes are similar in many respects. The lower part of Hildegard's Ecclesia and the actual wombs of normal women are both spaces for containing something related to life. Ecclesia receives and nurtures the floating souls inside her, as the normal womb accepts semen, grows an embryo with a soul, and nurtures it within its inner space. In Hildegard's vision, Ecclesia provides the sinful black souls with a process of rebirth by purifying them, or causing them to become white, and then setting them free. A normal woman grows a new human life in pregnancy and then "sets it free" through labour. These two processes are also related through their involvement of the mouth, through which Ecclesia sends out souls and through which mothers feed an embryo.

In addition, the salvational procedure of Ecclesia and the reproductive course of the womb are necessarily accompanied by physical pain. In *Scivias*, while Ecclesia cleanses the black souls by drawing them from her stomach to her mouth, Hildegard describes her as groaning. The salvational process is "the true ablution"[5] that allows Ecclesia to guide the souls to God. This purification is painful since the souls have to travel through her body from the bottom to the top. It goes without saying that even normal childbirth can be physically tortuous. It is well known that medieval childbirth was so dangerous that many women died in labour due to lack of nutritional and medical resources. In both cases, however, pain was treated as an essential part of accomplishing these female duties.

These similarities between Hildegard's vision of Ecclesia and the actual childbirth process point to Hildegard's view of the salvational or new-life-giving function of women. Hildegard's representation of the reproductive body does not evoke the inferior or degraded status of women. Rather, a woman's capacity for generation, labour, and maternal care is foregrounded and symbolizes the concrete operation of God's will to save people from sin and cleanse their souls for eternal life. This salvational process uses the woman's body as an important metaphor for the holiness of the entire dispensational process governed by God and for its material and immaterial parts working together.

---

5 Hildegard of Bingen, *Scivias*, trans. Hart and Bishop, 171; Hildegard of Bingen, *Scivias*, ed. Führkötter and Carelvaris, pt. 2, bk. 3, chap. 6, p. 139.

Although the direction of spiritual rebirth is opposite to that of actual childbirth, both processes signify a new birth. Hildegard's use of the female body has two positive aspects. First, the woman's body is not defiled but purifying. Hence, the physicality of the female reproductive organs and their specific processes become a metaphor for salvation. Second, the body of the woman is not simply a vessel that remains passive when it receives semen or while it allows the baby to develop. Rather, the womb has an ongoing and active role in purifying the woman's body. The womb is not just a passive place of containment; it is an active living organ with important work. For this reason alone, the womb also becomes an allegory of soul cleansing.

God's Maternal Love with Fluidity

Ecclesia's care for her children also does not end with birth but continues with the provision of both love and milk. God's divinity is fluid, and sometimes Ecclesia stands in as a figure of maternal love. But the imagery is very similar. God's maternal love is inherited by the Church, also the mother of believers in *Scivias*. Hildegard often uses the analogy of a mother's love, especially when describing unconditional love. The following passage from *Scivias* compares the Church's love to a mother's breast milk.

> And as a baby is nourished in its body by milk and the food another grinds up for it, so also a baptized person must observe from his inmost heart the doctrine and the faith given to him in his baptism. But if the baby does not suck at its mother's breast or take the food ground up for it, it will die at once; and so also if a baptized person does not receive the nurturing of his most loving mother, the Church, or retain the words his faithful teachers proposed to him at baptism, he will not escape a cruel death for his soul, for he has refused his soul's salvation and the sweetness of eternal life.[6]

---

6 Hildegard of Bingen, *Scivias*, trans. Hart and Bishop, 183. "Sed sicut infans de lacte et de escis ab alio sibi contritis corporaliter pascitur, ita etiam doctrinam et in baptismate sibi propositam fidem ex intimo corde obseruabit. Quod si ubera matris suae non sugit nec contritas sibi escas suscipit, incunctanter moritur, sic etiam si nutrimenta piissimae matris ecclesiae non accipit, nec uerba fidelium doctorum quae sibi in baptismate proposita sunt retinet, crudelitatem mortis animae non euadit; quoniam saluationem animae et dulcedinem aeternae uitae recusauit." Hildegard of Bingen, *Scivias*, ed. Führkötter and Carelvaris, pt. 2, bk. 2, chap. 33, p. 155.

Here, the Church's teaching regarding God is presented as being like milk, which even babies can swallow and digest without difficulty.[7] Babies, lacking teeth and having sensitive stomachs, cannot consume solid food like adults; they need milk or predigested ingredients. If they do not receive food in this way, they will die of hunger. Hildegard explains that the church's teachings are so soft and easily understood that even those who lack high intelligence or education can easily grasp them and so receive the benefits of salvation. God provides the Church as a means for humanity's survival. His teachings through the Church are conceived of here as a person's very first source of nourishment. Hildegard uses this analogy to foreground the motherly nature of God's love by emphasizing that he made the Church's teaching simple and basic so that anyone can receive it.

In her exegesis of Vision One in Book Two, when Hildegard presents God's process of creating humanity, she compares the mud moistened by God to a baby fed with mother's milk. As she describes the vision:

> Then the same flame was in that fire, and that burning extended itself to a little clod of mud which lay at the bottom of the atmosphere, and warmed it so that it was made flesh and blood, and blew upon it until it rose up a living human. When this was done, the blazing fire, by means of that flame which burned ardently with a gentle breath, offered to the human a white flower, which hung in that flame as dew hangs on the grass. Its scent came to the human's nostrils, but he did not taste it with his mouth or touch it with his hands and thus he turned away and fell into the thickest darkness, out of which he could not pull himself.[8]

---

7 Hildegard must have related this imagery to the milk and meat trope in the Pauline epistles, such as 1 Corinthians 3:2, "I have fed you with milk, and not with meat: for hitherto ye were not able to bear it, neither yet now are ye able," and Hebrews 5:12, "For when for the time ye ought to be teachers, ye have need that one teach you again which be the first principles of the oracles of God; and are become such as have need of milk, and not of strong meat."

8 Hildegard of Bingen, *Scivias*, trans. Hart and Bishop, 149. "Deinde etiam eadem flamma in igne et ardore illo extendit se ad paruam glebam limosae terrae iacentem in fundo eiusdem aeris eam calefaciens, ita quod caro et sanguis effecta est, eamque aspirans, ita quod uiuens homo erecta est. Quo facto ille lucidus ignis praebuit per eandem flammam leni flatu ardenter flagrantem ipsi homini candidissimum florem pendentem in eadem flamma ut ros pendet in gramine, cuius odorem idem homo naribus quidem sensit, sed gustum eius ore non percepit, nec manibus eum tetigit, ita uidelicet se auertens atque cadens in densissimas tenebras, de quibus se erigere non ualuit." Hildegard of Bingen, *Scivias*, ed. Führkötter and Carelvaris, pt. 2, bk. 1, p. 110.

Then Hildegard presents her readers with an exegesis.[9] The mud in this vision was at first weak and fragile, and it remained motionless until God heated it. Then, the body became flesh from the mud, and blood flowed through it. In order to fully become flesh, however, the mud still had to be nourished with moisture, which Hildegard compares to mother's milk. Or we might say that mother's milk enlivens a baby through nourishment, as God made mud into flesh through the animating power of heat. In this sense, both women's moisture and their milk, which are flows in their bodies, were understood as qualities with creative power.

Hildegard represents the woman's reproductive role through language that foregrounds God's provision of support and loving care.

> "And the children of those who afflicted you shall come and bow down to you, and all who slandered you shall worship your footsteps" [Isaiah 60:14]. What does this mean? O You Who are celestial Peace and the purest Sun. By You shall burst forth the living root, which is regeneration by the Spirit and water, and those who had lain prostrate under the heaviest curse in the filth of horrible impurity shall come eagerly to acknowledge You and thus bowed down, they will rise at last to truth and justice. How? They will suck the maternal sweetness of the true faith, not knowing it by sight but grasping it by faithful belief. And who are they? Those who sprang in sin from a race that never saw You in Your burning charity but persistently afflicted and oppressed You as if You were not their destined ruler; but who came to their senses and most sweetly loved You.[10]

---

9 Hildegard of Bingen, *Scivias*, trans. Hart and Bishop, 152. "Quod autem deinde eadem flamma in igne et ardore illo extendit se ad paruam glebam limosae terrae iacentem in fundo eiusdem aeris: hoc est quod creatis aliis creaturis Verbum Dei in forti uoluntate Patris et in amore supernae suauitatis inspexit pauperem et fragilem materiam mollis et tenacis fragilitatis humanitatis tam malorum quam bonorum procreandorum hominum in imo insensibilitatis et ponderositatis suae detentam et necdum acuto et uitali flatu excitatam; et eam calefaciens, ita quod caro et sanguis effecta est: id est in uiriditate calorem ei infundens, quoniam terra est carnalis materia hominis, nutriens eum suco suo sicut mater lactat filios suos; eamque aspirans ita quod uiuens homo erecta est: quia ipsam per supernam uirtutem excitauit atque in anima et corpore discernentem hominem mirabiliter eduxit." Hildegard of Bingen, *Scivias*, ed. Führkötter and Carelvaris, pt. 2, bk. 1, chap. 7, pp. 115–16.

10 Hildegard of Bingen, *Scivias*, trans. Hart and Bishop, 179. "*Et uenient ad te curui filii eorum qui humiliauerunt te, et adorabunt uestigia pedum tuorum omnes qui detrahebant tibi.* Quid est hoc? O tu, qui es superna pax et purissimus sol, per te ebulliet uiuens radix, quae est regeneratio Spiritus et aquae, cum illi sollerter uenient ad agnitionem tuam qui in spurcitia nefandissimae immunditiae sub grauissima maledictione prostrati erant: quoniam ipsi hoc modo quasi curui uix tandem ad ueritatem et ad iustitiam surgent. Quomodo? Ipse maternam dulcedinem uerae fidei sugent, eam uisibiliter uidendo nescientes, sed tantum illam fideliter

In this passage, Hildegard provides readers with her exegesis of a portion of Isaiah. She presents this passage as signifying how people were to come back to God from their sinful life. Although God was betrayed by his own creatures, he still loves them. Hildegard thus describes his love as maternal. As mothers feed their babies with milk, God feeds them with the "maternal sweetness of the true faith." According to Hildegard, the unconditional love of God is like a mother's love because God loves all his children, even the sinners, as a mother loves her children. Also, human beings suck in God's love without knowing what it is, as babies suck in their mothers' milk even though they do not intellectually understand what it is.

The Porous Womb, the Sealed Womb

There are certainly differences between Ecclesia and real women regarding the giving of life. Normal women were not considered "intact" after intercourse and childbirth, but Hildegard emphasizes that Ecclesia is still intact although she constantly draws in and emits souls through her body. In her virginity, she is linked to Mary. Hildegard relates Ecclesia's breasts glowing red to the heart of the Virgin Mary glowing with fiery devotion; both are to be praised, "like the dawn, greatly sparkling," for their virginity.[11] There is again a further exegesis of this vision in which Hildegard explains how Ecclesia's virgin body represents the wholeness of the Church:

> *But she groans, drawing them upward to her head, and they go out by her mouth, while she remains untouched.* For this blessed mother sighs inwardly when baptism is celebrated by the sacred anointing of the Holy Spirit, because the person is renewed by the true circumcision of the Spirit and water, and thus offered to the Supreme Beatitude Who is the Head of all, and made a member of Christ, regenerated unto salvation by invocation of the Holy Trinity. But in this that mother suffers no hurt, for she will remain for-

---

credendo rapentes. Et qui sunt illi? Videlicet isti qui in materia peccati de his orti qui te in ardenti caritate numquam uiderunt, sed qui te crudeliter opprimendo pertinaciter afflixerunt quasi tu illorum non dominareris, te in bono sensu dulcissime amauerunt." Hildegard of Bingen, *Scivias*, ed. Führkötter and Carelvaris, pt. 2, bk. 3, chap. 25, pp. 149–50.

11 Hildegard of Bingen, *Scivias*, trans. Hart and Bishop, 172. "In pectore eius uelut aurora rubeo fulgore rutilante: quia in cordibus fidelium integritas beatissimae Virginis Filium Dei generantis ardentissima deuotione fulget, ubi etiam multimodo genere musicorum audis de ipsa 'quasi aurora ualde rutilans' decantari: quoniam omnis uox credentium, ut intellectui tuo infunditur, uirginitatem eiusdem illibatae Virginis tota intentione in ecclesia amplecti debet." Hildegard of Bingen, *Scivias*, ed. Führkötter and Carelvaris, pt. 2, bk. 3, chap. 9, p. 140.

> ever in the wholeness of virginity, which is the Catholic faith; for she arose in the blood of the true Lamb, her intimate Bridegroom, Who was born of the untouched Virgin without any corruption of integrity. So too that Bride will remain untouched, so that no schism can corrupt her.[12]

For Hildegard, Ecclesia's virginity is not just about physical or spiritual integrity. Her unbroken body demonstrates the unbrokenness of the Catholic Church, just as Mary was the virginal mother of the Saviour.[13] Hildegard equates Ecclesia with the Virgin Mary and Ecclesia's giving birth to cleansed souls with Mary's giving birth to Jesus. This means not only that Ecclesia has to remain virginal like the Virgin Mary, but also that both virginal bodies serve as symbols of the integrity of the Church.

While schisms have been viewed as deeply problematic throughout Christian history, maintaining the unity of the Church was of special importance in Hildegard of Bingen's time. The importance of Church unity was often emphasized through symbolic representations, mystical interpretations, and biblical exegesis, which all appear in Hildegard's writings. In the period of Hildegard's lifetime, the Church experienced major ruptures, such as the East–West Schism of 1054, earlier in the century of her birth, the effects of which continued to shape the ecclesiastical climate she inhabited. Her era also saw numerous papal resignations, with twenty-four popes elected and stepping down, though not all were considered legitimate. Among them,

---

12 Hildegard of Bingen, *Scivias*, trans. Hart and Bishop, 173. "Vnde et illa ingemit, sursum eos ad caput suum trahens, ubi ad os eius exeunt, ipsa tamen integra permanente: quoniam haec beata mater intima suspiria trahit, quando baptisma cum chrismate in sanctificatione Spiritus sancti consecratur, cum homo in uera circumcisione Spiritus et aquae innouandus est, ita illo summae beatitudini, quae caput omnium est, oblato et membro Christi facto, cum per inuocationem sanctae Trinitatis quasi per os beatae matris ad saluationem regeneratur, nullam laesionem eadem matre patiente, quia ipsa in aeternum permanebit in integritate uirginitatis suae, quae fides catholica est; quoniam exorta est in sanguine ueri agni uidelicet intimi sponsi sui, qui sine ulla corruptione integritatis ex integerrima Virgine natus est. Sic et eadem sponsa integra permanebit, ita quod nullum schisma eam corrumpere poterit." Hildegard of Bingen, *Scivias*, ed. Führkötter and Carelvaris, pt. 2, bk. 3, chap. 12, pp. 141–42.

13 Hildegard of Bingen, *Scivias*, trans. Hart and Bishop, 173–74. "Vnde et ecclesia omnium Christianorum uirginea mater est; quoniam in secreto Spiritus sancti eos concipit et parit, illos Deo offerens, ita quod et filii Dei uocantur. Et ut beatam Matrem Spiritus sanctus obumbrauit, ita quod sine dolore mirabiliter Filium Dei concepit et peperit et tamen uirgo permansit, sic et ecclesiam felicem matrem credentium Spiritus sanctus illustrat, ita quod sine ulla corruptione simpliciter filios concipit et parit et uirgo perdurat. Quid est hoc?" Hildegard of Bingen, *Scivias*, ed. Führkötter and Carelvaris, pt. 2, bk. 3, chap. 12, p. 142.

Hildegard particularly criticized the papal schism of 1130–1138 following the death of Pope Honorius II, when two popes were appointed and created confusion in religion and politics.[14] Hildegard of Bingen advocated for Church reform. She perceived that the Church and its male authorities were not fulfilling their responsibilities adequately.[15] As noted above, this led her to characterize her era as "effeminate," and she did not hesitate to critique male clergy not for being "manly" enough. Her visions of Ecclesia, on the other hand, highlighted its integrity, just like that of the Virgin Mary.

Not only did Hildegard warn about schismatic tribulations in her lifetime through her writings, but she was also later regarded as one of the major apocalyptic figures who foresaw the coming ecclesiastical divisions. Later, her works gained particular relevance during the Western Schism (1378–1417), underscoring her enduring importance in Church history and her role in advocating for ecclesiastical reform.[16]

Imperfection and Wounds Enabling Flows

At the same time, however, in Hildegard's vision, openings and flows are integral parts of Ecclesia. Her body is not closed off or sealed like the ideal female body of the Virgin Mary. Hildegard highly valued the virginal body of women and understood sexual experience as rupture or a higher degree of openness.[17] These open features of Ecclesia might be viewed as inferior and incomplete. Nevertheless, they allow her to receive, purge, and release sinful

---

14 For more information regarding the papacy in Hildegard's time, see Corrigan, "Hildegard of Bingen," 359–61.

15 This criticism of the Church was picked up by Pope Benedict XVI in a General Audience Address in 2010. The pope used her allegory of the open wounds of Jesus in criticizing the clergy's response to child abuse among the priesthood. Campbell, "The Prophetess and the Pope," 23–24.

16 Magda Hayton has closely examined how Hildegard was incorporated into the apocalyptic traditions of late medieval France. See Hayton, "Hildegardian Prophecy and French Prophecy Collections," 453–91.

17 Hildegard praises virginal women: "O dearest seeds, O flowers sweeter and more exquisite than any perfumes, whose soft fragility rises like the dawn to betrothal with my Son, loving Him dearly with chaste love, she is His bride and He is her Bridegroom, for this race of virgins loves Him dearly and so is to be adorned in the Heavenly Kingdom with glorious ornaments!" Hildegard of Bingen, *Scivias*, trans. Hart and Bishop, 178. "O carissima germina et o dulciores et suauiores flores super omnia aromata, ubi mollis et fragilis natura quasi aurora ad desponsationem Filii mei consurgit, casta dilectione ualde amans eum, ipsa scilicet ei sponsa et ipse illi sponsus, cum hoc genus uirginum ualde diligit eum in superno regno insignibus

souls. Ecclesia's imperfection enabled her to save humankind, although it caused her to suffer in the fight against evil.

A woman's body, compared to a man's body, is weaker in Hildegard's religious and medical accounts and thus is often understood as imperfect. Eve was created out of Adam's flesh, having the softer and weaker body. Eve was already breakable and permeable to sin, which we see through her being tempted and deceived first by evil. What is even worse, Eve's original sin made her body open to flux, such as menstrual flow and the reproductive process. The perforated bodies of women and the flow of blood and childbirth were used to support belief in the weakness of women.

However, as I have already discussed, the less perfect bodies of Eve and women helped them to avoid the aftermath of original sin. And this imperfection allows women to menstruate, thereby purging their bodies and having babies through their porous wombs. Unlike the man's body, which is relatively more closed up and solid, the woman's weakness opens the gate to reproduction through her own body. Likewise, Ecclesia, which of course has a female body, is imperfect in order to become perfected and then elevated to Jerusalem. The wounds and pain caused by Ecclesia's flawed body are what make her unimpaired as the bride of Christ and the mother of Christ's offspring. Through her maternal compassion in saving souls with her imperfect body, Ecclesia ultimately becomes the mother who bears Christ's spiritual children.

In the exegesis of her mystical experience, Hildegard explains the image of Ecclesia as the manifestation of God's love. She interprets Ecclesia as having "maternal" kindness. The many holes in her belly allow Ecclesia to capture as many fish-like souls as possible in order to save them, recalling Jesus's analogy between fishing and his own salvational role as a process of making his followers "fishers of men" in Matthew 4:19. Ecclesia shares this duty with the followers of Jesus. Ecclesia's womb is perforated with many holes so that it can catch as many souls as she can. Now, Ecclesia can accomplish Jesus's role as a net catching fish.[18]

---

ornamentis uidelicet adornandum!" Hildegard of Bingen, *Scivias*, ed. Führkötter and Carelvaris, pt. 2, bk. 3, chap. 23, p. 148.

18 Hildegard of Bingen, *Scivias*, trans. Hart and Bishop, 171. "Quod autem uenter eius est in modum retis perforatus multis foraminibus, in quibus maxima multitudo hominum discurrit: hoc est materna benignitas ipsius quae ad capturam fidelium animarum perspicua est diuerso acumine uirtutum, in quibus credentes populi per fidem uerae credulitatis deuote conuersantur. Sed is qui rete suum proiecit in capturam piscium est Filius meus, sponsus dilectae ecclesiae suae, quam in cruore

Hildegard even suggests that Ecclesia needs to endure more pain to gain perfection in the future. According to her, Ecclesia in her vision is not perfect, which is manifested as the body without legs or feet. Her imperfection lets her suffer on the last day of the world, "when the son of perdition comes to delude the world." However, Ecclesia's "bleeding" wounds from her battles against evil will accomplish her perfection. With this perfection, Ecclesia is reborn through the blood of Jesus as a new bride in Jerusalem.[19] And this scene reminds readers of how Jesus as Christ came to the world. In Christian theology, he came to the world, suffered, and was killed in a human body, which was degenerate and perishable due to Adam's transgressions. When Jesus's weak point was mortality, however, it was death that made Jesus perfect. Through his death, he was able to sacrifice himself in order to save humankind from their evil deeds.

In Hildegard's vision of the foreseen Last Judgement, blood is again emphasized and signifies the suffering of both Ecclesia and Jesus.[20] Ecclesia bleeds from evil's attack on the Last Day; Jesus shed blood in his sacrifice. Additionally, Ecclesia is perfected through the shedding of her blood, while Jesus accomplished his salvational role in his crucifixion, when he shed blood from his side, as vividly depicted in medieval paintings. Just like Jesus's death, the process of Ecclesia painfully purifying souls is a sacrificial act. As human beings constantly sin, Ecclesia continually suffers, which Hildegard explains as "the sweetest sacrifice."[21] Through endless labour, she continues to perfect the heavenly plan to save people. However, this is not the only pain she will endure. Hildegard foresees that more suffering awaits

---

suo sibi desponsauit ad reparandum casum perditi hominis." Hildegard of Bingen, *Scivias*, ed. Führkötter and Carelvaris, pt. 2, bk. 3, chap. 4, p. 138.

19 Hildegard of Bingen, *Scivias*, trans. Hart and Bishop, 171. "Quae nondum crura aut pedes habet: quia nondum ad fortitudinem constantiae suae, nec ad candorem completionis suae perducta est; quoniam circa tempus filii perditionis, qui mundo errorem inducet, igneam et sanguineam crudelissimae peruersitatis angustiam plenissime in membris suis patietur, per quam calamitatem in sanguineis uulneribus ad perfectum perducta propere currat in caelestem Ierusalem, cum etiam in sanguine Filii mei noua nupta suauiter exorta est, ipsa hoc ardore intrans uitam in plenitudine gaudii subolis suae." Hildegard of Bingen, *Scivias*, ed. Führkötter and Carelvaris, pt. 2, bk. 3, chap. 5, p. 138.

20 In a study focused on a period much later than Hildegard's time, Bynum points out that devotion to Jesus's blood flourished in Northern Europe especially during the fourteenth and fifteenth centuries. Bynum, *Wonderful Blood*, 6.

21 Hildegard of Bingen, *Scivias*, trans. Hart and Bishop, 171; Hildegard of Bingen, *Scivias*, ed. Führkötter and Carelvaris, pt. 2, bk. 3, chap. 6, p. 139.

Ecclesia, but that it will make her perfect—a perfection through suffering which is described in Hildegard's Book Three.

The Sun, Moon, and Stars in Flows

For Hildegard, flow is important in salvation and happens in and through Ecclesia's body. In the time before Noah, God had to destroy the world to cleanse it because there was no way to create a flow of penance that could match the flow of sin. People did not repent or ask for forgiveness from God. They were moving in one direction—away from God—by sinning and could not return themselves back to God. In this way, humanity failed to complete the cyclical flow, which was why they were killed by God's judgment to cleanse all the filth from the world. However, according to Hildegard, Jesus enabled a more consistent flow of souls back to God. God did not need to repeat this mass killing once he sent Jesus into the world through the virginal womb of Mary and instituted the sacraments of the Church as a means of continuous purgation of sin to complete the cycle.

In Vision Five of Book Two, Hildegard describes the church as having a cycle itself in the form of the three orders of the church, monasticism, priesthood, and secular life, which operate according to a hierarchy. Hildegard uses the celestial system to explain the salvational economy, as each part makes circular movements. According to Hildegard, there is a hierarchy among the sun, moon, and stars. The sun is Jesus, who flows from the heart of God to the womb of the Virgin Mary. He illuminates the world. Flow is emphasized once again, as the sun makes its way from sunrise to sunset, and its light appears and disappears as it follows its daily course. The moon represents Ecclesia, betrothed to Jesus, the sun. The Church and the moon flow through waxing and waning, which Hildegard calls "a cycle of movement." Unlike the sun and Jesus, the moon and the Church do not have a blazing light. Instead, Jesus and the Church have complementary roles just as the sun and moon do; when the sun and Jesus shine, the moon and the Church do not illuminate. But when the sun and Jesus are not present in this world, as at night, the moon and Ecclesia receive their salvational roles, although the impact might be milder. In this "cycle of movement," the Church inflates with more children and deflates with fewer children depending on the increase of virtue or evil. Ecclesia could suffer and be harmed by malicious people, whom Hildegard refers to as bad Christians, Jews, or pagans. However, Ecclesia will continue to shine because her light is coming through Jesus from God, similar to the moon receiving its source of light from the sun. Finally, there are the stars, in the lowest position in this celestial order. The stars are religious people who have joined the orders of the Church.

> These are great mysteries. For consider the sun and the moon and the stars. I formed the sun to give light by day, and the moon and stars to give light by night. The sun symbolizes My Son, Who went forth from My heart and illuminated the world when in the latest times He was born of the Virgin, as the sun goes forth and lights the world when it rises at the end of the night. And the moon symbolizes the Church, betrothed to My Son in true and celestial betrothal. And the moon is so made that it always increases and decreases, but does not burn of itself unless it is kindled by the light of the sun, so too the Church has a cycle of movement: her children sometimes rise in increase of virtues and sometimes decline by inconstant behavior or harm by outside forces. For she is often assailed in her mysteries by ravening wolves, that is to say malicious people, whether bad Christians or Jews or pagans; and she is not fired to endurance by herself, but lit up by Me through My Son to persevere in good. But the stars, which differ from each other in the brightness of their glory, symbolize the people in the differing religious orders of the Church.[22]

In this vision, which alludes to 1 Corinthians 15, God tells Hildegard that Jesus is like the sun, the Church like the moon, and people like the stars. In 1 Corinthians 15:40–42—"There are bodies celestial and bodies terrestrial: but, one is the glory of the celestial, and another of the terrestrial. One is the glory of the sun, another the glory of the moon, and another the glory of the stars. For star differeth from star in glory. So also is the resurrection of the dead. It is sown in corruption: it shall rise in incorruption"—the sun, moon, and stars are all compared to different kinds of people.

---

22 Hildegard of Bingen, *Scivias*, trans. Hart and Bishop, 202. "Magna mysteria sunt haec. Considera enim solem et lunam et stellas. Ego formaui solem ut luceat in die et lunam et stellas ut luceant in nocte. Sol autem significat Filium meum, qui de corde meo exiuit et mundum illuminauit cum natus est ex Virgine in fine temporum, sicut et sol egrediens mundum illustrat cum oritur circa finem noctis. Sed luna ecclesiam eidem Filio meo in uera et superna desponsatione desponsatam designat. Et ut luna semper incrementum et defectum in sua constitutione habet, sed a se ipsa non ardet nisi quod a lumine solis incenditur, sic et ecclesia in circuitione motionis est, ita quod filii eius saepe proficiunt in incremento uirtutum, et quod saepe deficient in diuersitate morum atque in dispersione aduersitatum, ita quod multoties in mysteriis suis per rapacissimos lupos impugnatur, uidelicet per malignos homines tam malorum Christianorum quam Iudaeorum et paganorum, et in hoc per semetipsam ad tolerantiam non accenditur, sed in me per Filium meum ut in bono perseueret illuminatur. Stellae autem a se differentes in claritate fulgoris sui significant populum diuersi ordinis ecclesiasticae religionis." Hildegard of Bingen, *Scivias*, ed. Führkötter and Carelvaris, pt. 2, bk. 5, pp. 176–77.

Hildegard builds on this comparison: In the beginning Jesus is identified with the sun because of his strong power to shine, and at the end, the stars are interpreted as the religious orders. In the middle, the Church is thought of as the moon, because the moon reflects the sun's light and because of its cyclical movement. Hildegard connects the waxing of the moon to the good deeds of Christians: if people follow what God commands, the church will wax like the moon. By contrast, if people commit sin through bad behaviour or by denying Christ as the Jews or pagans did, the Church will wane just like the moon. The moon is an important symbol because its changes in size are visible; it is the only celestial body with visible phases, waxing and waning.

While Hildegard does not comment on this, it is interesting how the identification of Ecclesia with the moon adds another feminine dimension to Ecclesia. The association emphasizes their cyclical nature: Ecclesia, like the moon, increases and decreases as the number of good Christians changes. The Church goes through its own cycle by receiving a flow of good Christians and expelling a flow of "malicious" Christians and nonbelievers. Implicitly, this cyclical process is meant to resemble how the human body keeps its balance.

The Woman's Body is Open to Purge and Therefore Save People

The vision of Ecclesia in *Scivias* shows how Hildegard uses the female body and a woman's reproductive process to illustrate how God's salvation works. While Hildegard is fully in line with the traditional depictions of Ecclesia here, she interestingly presents the detailed steps of a process through which the female body of Ecclesia could cleanse and save people. She intentionally adapts images of childbirth and purgation which are presumably drawn from her medical knowledge of gynaecological practices. An important feature of this complexity of roles and representations of femininity is the understanding of flow.

In *Scivias*, it is clear that Hildegard attaches religious importance to flow. As we have seen in her *Cause et cure*, Hildegard appreciates the medical importance of bodily flow as a key method of keeping the body in balance. The human body, in this view, communicates with the world by receiving needed elements and expelling superfluous materials. Viewing it as an expulsion of superfluous materials, Hildegard presents a positive view of menstruation; it is the way in which the female body cleanses itself through its openness. Likewise, Hildegard believes that flow is essential for human salvation. In *Scivias*, holy flow could signify the movement of divinity into matter, as when Jesus descends from heaven into the womb of the Virgin Mary. Flow could also signify purgation, as in the washing away of sin. Women's bodies, characterized by greater porosity in Hildegard's and other medieval medical understandings, served as ideal vessels for facilitating this essential flow not only in physical ways but also in spiritual ways.

Ecclesia's cleansing is connected to baptism and the flow of water. Hildegard continues to emphasize baptism in *Scivias* as a replacement for circumcision. She explains the process of Ecclesia's purgation as the fountain of baptism. While circumcision was the custom of the patriarchs, baptism is the new treatment for the sinful.[23] The physical covenant of circumcision was replaced by Jesus's "true font of baptism" when he came to the world. At the same time, baptism is akin to a weapon that people can use to protect themselves.

The font and the pouring of water vivify not only human beings but Jesus as well. According to Hildegard, divine power created Jesus's body, and the Holy Spirit brought his soul to life "by the pouring out of water" like other human beings.

> It receives into Itself the spirit of the person, restoring him to life, as he is first brought into life on a wave of blood when he comes out of the vessel of the body. And just as a human form is then lovingly formed and called human, so now the soul of the person is vivified in water before the eyes of God, so that God knows that he is an inheritor of life.[24]

Hildegard continues that baptism is open to everyone regardless of their age or sex. While circumcision is limited to men and predominantly performed for a certain age group, baptism can be performed for any gender and is not

---

23 Hildegard of Bingen, *Scivias*, trans. Hart and Bishop, 175. "Nam duo signa legis signatorum tradita noscuntur hominibus, scilicet circumcisio in antiquis patribus et baptismus in nouis doctoribus, per quae iugati sunt homines ut bos iugo suo; quoniam quamuis ille stimulo corriperetur, tamen curuum sulcum faceret, si iugo ligatus non esset." Hildegard of Bingen, *Scivias*, ed. Führkötter and Carelvaris, pt. 2, bk. 3, chap. 16, pp. 144–45.

24 Hildegard of Bingen, *Scivias*, trans. Hart and Bishop, 181–82. "Ita quod homo per illud in regeneratione uiuit. Nam sicut homo nascitur ex carne, diuina potestate in forma Adae illum creante, ita Spiritus sanctus recuperat uitam animae per inundationem aquae, cum ipsa spiritum hominis in se accipit eum resuscitans ad uitam, ut prius in unda sanguinis suscitatus est, cum in corporali uasculo manifestatus est. Vt enim forma hominis tunc amabiliter formatur, ita quod homo dicitur, sic spiritus hominis ante oculos Dei nunc in aqua uiuificatur, ita quod eum Deus ad hereditatem uitae nouit." Hildegard of Bingen, *Scivias*, ed. Führkötter and Carelvaris, pt. 2, bk. 3, chap. 30, p. 153.

limited to any age group. Of course, baptism is accessible to women, including Hildegard of Bingen herself.

Hildegard describes Ecclesia giving birth to souls in Book Three of *Scivias*. In the same vision, Hildegard explains that a salvational flow courses through Ecclesia's body:

> *And the children who have passed through the womb of the image walk in the splendor that surrounds her*; which means that they, who through the font of sacred baptism have the Church as their happy mother, should remain in and keep to the divine law by which that mother is illuminated and adorned, for if they renounce it by infidelity they will again be stained by the sins from which they had been cleansed.[25]

Here, Hildegard comments on the children who have passed through Ecclesia's womb and are walking in "the splendor that surrounds her." She interprets this "splendor" as the divine law by which Ecclesia is illuminated. This law is meant to be followed by the baptized congregation; implicitly, if too many people failed to obey the law, their mother Church would lose her illumination. Thus, to maintain the illuminating law of the Church, people must continually flow into her body, where they are cleansed and then returned. The flow of people into the Church enables the mother's divine light to stay alive. Ecclesia is the everlasting flow of a cleansing fountain inasmuch as she is able to repeatedly purify any sinner. At least three kinds of flow overlap here: the flow of people, of the Church's divine illumination, and of the Church's cleansing grace. If any one of these flows stopped, the whole process would collapse.

The flow is important and should be continuous. According to Hildegard, human beings corrupt themselves by committing sin again and again while they are alive. Therefore, if any person wants to go to Heaven, they should be revived through baptism or "water and the Spirit," as John 3:5 says in the New Testament.[26] Why? Hildegard traces the problem back to the first human beings who committed the original sin. Human beings are already

---

25 Hildegard of Bingen, *Scivias*, trans. Hart and Bishop, 175. "Sed quod infantes qui uentrem praedictae imaginis transierant in splendore qui eam circumdederat ambulant: hoc est quod hi quorum mater felix ecclesia per fontem sacri baptismatis exsistit, in lege diuina, qua eadem mater illustrata et ornata est, permanere atque eam conseruare debent, ne si eam infideliter abiecerint, rursum peccatis a quibus mundati erant inquinentur." Hildegard of Bingen, *Scivias*, ed. Führkötter and Carelvaris, pt. 2, bk. 3, chap. 14, p. 144.

26 "Truly, truly I say to you, unless a man is born again of water and the Spirit, he cannot enter the Kingdom of Heaven."

polluted when they are born due to "burning heat" and "a poisonous form."[27] Here, it is interesting that both heat and poison are more closely linked to Adam, as Hildegard's *Cause et cure* explains. It is the woman, the Virgin Mary, who makes it possible for human beings to be cleansed by "the water of sanctification and the spirit of illumination" from innate sin.

For Hildegard, human beings are to be enlivened twice. When they are conceived and while they develop in their mother's womb, they are to have a soul poured into them. And in order to achieve salvation, they must have spirit poured into them through baptism. For Hildegard, reproduction is also purification. The poisonous semen that originated from Adam is nullified and heated in the womb. Baptism gives people the "birth of joy." Both processes are purifying; while birth is to be cleansed from original sin, rebirth is from the sin that people constantly commit.

Hildegard explains sanctification in terms of cleansing flows. She suggests that people flow in spirit, like water, by nature. Her thought process then turns to the water of baptism. Just as dirt is cleansed by water and spirit animates lifeless matter, humans need to be reborn in water and spirit before they are accepted into Heaven. The human spirit's watery nature reflects the divine flow. As with the symbolic connection between the flood's enormous cleansing power and the advent of Christ above, humanity itself is depicted as an image of the flow of "enlivening" spirit (*spiritus vegetationis*)—a flow that merges with baptismal purging in this passage, which is closely connected to Hildegard's emphasis on *viriditas*. In this way, Hildegard identifies

---

27 "With firmest certainty and not with wavering doubt, I say to you who are born of filth that Man, risen out of burning heat and wrapped in a poisonous form, will be confounded by his apathy unless in the true joy of a new child he is born again from the water of sanctification and the spirit of illumination. How? Because Man, who overflows like water with the spirit of his enlivening, will not be able to enter into salvation as an heir to the Kingdom of his Creator unless he is purified by the true regeneration, as water cleans the dirty and spirit gives life to the inanimate; for he is guilty of the sin of the first parent, who was fraudulently deceived by the Devil." Hildegard of Bingen, *Scivias*, trans. Hart and Bishop, 180. "*Amen, amen, dico tibi, nisi quis renatus fuerit ex aqua et Spiritu, non potest introire in regnum Dei*. Quid est hoc? Constantissima certitudine et non instabili ambiguitate dico tibi, qui natus es ex putredine, quia homo qui exortus est de ardenti calore et inuolutus uenenosae facturae, nisi in uero gaudio nouae subolis renascatur ex aqua sanctificationis et Spiritu illuminationis, in tepore neglectus sui confunditur. Quomodo? Quia homo uelut aqua cum spiritu uegetationis suae inundans, quoniam ut aqua sordes emundat et ut spiritus inanimata uiuificat, nisi in uera regeneratione purgetur, non poterit per introitum saluationis heres regni creatoris sui fieri; quia in peccato primi parentis quem diabolus fraudulenter decepit obligatus est." Hildegard of Bingen, *Scivias*, ed. Führkötter and Carelvaris, pt. 2, bk. 3, chap. 27, p. 151.

the flow that sustains earthly life with the process of purification that leads to everlasting life. The flow must continue to advance God's design.

In another vision, Hildegard sees the same children who have passed through Ecclesia's womb and observes that some now seem healthier than others:

> And I saw those children who, as mentioned before, had passed through the womb of that image, shining with great brightness; some of them were adorned with gold color from their foreheads to their feet, but others lacked that color and had only the brightness....Of those who were meditating on the pure and brilliant splendor, some had clear eyes and strong feet and were marching forward vigorously in the womb of the image; but others had weak eyes and crippled feet and were blown here and there by the wind.[28]

Like the previous vision, this Vision Four of Book Two represents souls as children and Ecclesia as a female body able to wash away their sins. Here, the souls are distinguished according to their merits. Those who are described with "healthier" features, such as clear eyes and strong feet, voluntarily enter the church (the womb of Ecclesia) to do penance and be purified. On the other hand, the souls with "weaker" bodies, which can be seen as disabilities, merely return to the same place. In the sixth exegesis of this vision, Hildegard says:

> *And you see those children who, as mentioned before, had passed through the womb of that image, shining with great brightness.* These are they who in the innocence of a clean and pure heart have gained a mother, the Church, in the font of regeneration, as was shown to you before, and are children of light, for their sins are washed away.[29]

There are also children, or souls, who never undergo the process of penance and purification. Whether they have clear or weak eyes and strong or

28 Hildegard of Bingen, *Scivias*, trans. Hart and Bishop, 189. "Et infantes illos qui uentrem eiusdem imaginis, ut praedictum est, transierant uidi multa claritate fulgentes...Sed ex his qui ipsum purum et lucidum splendorem considerabant quidam claros oculos et fortes pedes habebant ac in uentre eiusdem imaginis fortiter incedebant. Alii autem infirmos oculos et debiles pedes habentes huc et illuc a uento proiciebantur." Hildegard of Bingen, *Scivias*, ed. Führkötter and Carelvaris, pt. 2, bk. 4, p. 160.

29 Hildegard of Bingen, *Scivias*, trans. Hart and Bishop, 192. "Et quod uides infantes illos qui uentrem eiusdem imaginis, ut praedictum est, transierant, multa claritate fulgentes: hoc est quod hi qui in innocentia munditiae puri cordis per fontem regenerationis matrem scilicet ecclesiam, ut tibi praemonstratum est, adepti sunt, filii lucis propter ablutionem peccatorum suorum exsistunt." Hildegard of Bingen, *Scivias*, ed. Führkötter and Carelvaris, pt. 2, bk. 4, chap. 6, p. 164.

weak feet, some children succeed in bringing themselves in front of Ecclesia so that they can touch her. However, others do not approach Ecclesia and are left "in the elation of the way of death."[30] In this vision, then, Hildegard emphasizes the cleansing function of Ecclesia's female body for the sake of humanity's salvation. In whatsoever manner, once children enter Ecclesia's womb, they are cleansed and saved.

This emphasis on flow appears again in Vision Four of Book Two, where Hildegard explains her unique vision of confirmation in Mother Church. Here, Ecclesia stands before a white tower, which signifies "the flaming forth of the gifts of the Holy Spirit."[31] It seems that Hildegard views Ecclesia as being supported by the Holy Spirit, which protects her against evil as a tower defends a city.[32]

Hildegard also relates Ecclesia's duty through baptism as purification through a reference to Hebrew scripture. Referring to 2 Kings 1:23, "The King went over the brook of Cedron, and all the people marched toward the way of the olive trees, which led to the desert," she interprets the sentence about the king crossing the brook as signifying the baptism of Christ. Hildegard contrasts "the flowing waters of the blessed washing" to "the desert of Adam's sin." According to Hildegard, Jesus brought salvation and thus provided ever-flowing water to people who would have wandered in the desert because of their original sin. Flow is as important in anointing as in baptism and salvation.[33]

---

30 Hildegard of Bingen, *Scivias*, trans. Hart and Bishop, 189. Hildegard of Bingen, *Scivias*, ed. Führkötter and Carelvaris, pt. 2, bk. 4, chap. 30, p. 160.

31 Hildegard of Bingen, *Scivias*, trans. Hart and Bishop, 190. "Flagrationem donorum Spiritus sancti." Hildegard of Bingen, *Scivias*, ed. Führkötter and Carelvaris, pt. 2, bk. 4, chap. 1, p. 161.

32 Hildegard of Bingen, *Scivias*, trans. Hart and Bishop, 191. "Quia Spiritus sanctus in maxima fortitudine incarnationis illius qui uerus sponsus ecclesiae exsistit mirabilia sua mirabiliter operatus est, et ecclesiam tam fortem in defensione munitionis suae ostendit, quod ita prae fortitudine illa sua ab igneo dono eius munita est numquam in errore ullius peruersitatis deici poterit; quoniam per supernam protectionem in amore sponsi sui sine macula et sine ruga semper gaudebit, quia et idem Vnigenitus meus de Spiritu sancto conceptus nobiliter sine macula ex Virgine natus est, quemadmodum ad Moysen locutus sum." Hildegard of Bingen, *Scivias*, ed. Führkötter and Carelvaris, pt. 2, bk. 4, chap. 4, p. 163.

33 Hildegard of Bingen, *Scivias*, trans. Hart and Bishop, 192–93. "*Rex quoque transgrediebatur torrentem Cedron, et cunctus populus incedebat contra uiam oliuae, quae respiciebat ad desertum.* Quid est hoc? Filius Virginis, qui dominatur uniuerso mundo ut rex terrenus reliquo populo, transgressus est torrentes aquas beati lauacri, quod in admonitione Spiritus sancti forti desiderio uiam salutis demonstrat. Quid

In *Scivias*, Hildegard emphasizes the importance of keeping the flow of repentance ongoing to fully atone for one's sin. In her view, human beings are bound to commit sin repeatedly. After Adam committed his first sin, people became so weak in body and spirit that they were easily distracted by evil temptation, like those children with weaker bodies who were easily blown away. However, according to Hildegard, people would be saved as long as they recognized and continually repented for their faults. God would accept them whenever they returned to him because he loves them as his children. In this sense, Hildegard's theology emphasizes the significance of flow to both the commission and the purgation of sin. Just as women have to menstruate in order to purge superfluous fluids, Christians have to take action to return to God because they frequently make mistakes.

For Hildegard, flow encompasses women's roles in reproductive processes. Constant flows are represented through menstruation, conception, lactation, and childbirth. And the same flow vividly characterizes God's salvational plan through Ecclesia. While Hildegard of Bingen sees Ecclesia as having a female body, especially a womb, Ecclesia's main role is to receive people who have sinned and send out them cleansed in a constant circle. This process is not dissimilar to a woman's purgative menstruation and reproduction, which is possible due to the woman's porous body, not the man's relatively closed body. Furthermore, this is why the Virgin Mary could receive the Holy Spirit into her womb and send Jesus into the world.

Through her portrayal of Ecclesia, Hildegard directly bridges medical concepts of childbirth and bodily flow with theological visions of salvation in *Scivias*. The perforated womb that receives, transforms, and releases souls parallels the physiological functions she describes in *Cause et cure*. Hildegard thus affirms that the physiological porosity of women's bodies serves as both metaphor and mechanism for spiritual renewal, elevating medical knowledge to salvational significance.

---

est hoc? Ipse reliquit mortem transiens ad uitam, cum in regeneratione Spiritus et aquae, id est in magno ornamento urbis caelestis Ierusalem, quae numquam deficit, summam beatitudinem enuntiauit. Vnde omnis populus qui in illum credebat iuit per inspirationem sancti Spiritus ad uiam illam quae absconsa erat, in unctione olei respicientis ad praeuaricationem Adae, quae deserta erat pulchritudine hereditatis iustitiae Dei, et considerantis utrum illa ad salutem redire uellet an non: quia uulneratum peccatum primi hominis necesse habuit ut per sacerdotale officium inungeretur, quod Filio Virginis necesse non erat, quoniam ipse totus in sanctitate conceptus est, non uulnerato nec corrupto Matris suae utero, sed in integritatis honore perseuerante." Hildegard of Bingen, *Scivias*, ed. Führkötter and Carelvaris, pt. 2, bk. 4, chap. 7, p. 165.

Afterword

ALTERNATIVE MEDICINE

FROM OLD KNOWLEDGE TO NEW PRACTICE THROUGH THE WOMAN'S BODY

THE POROSITY OF the woman's body is not only found in medieval Western medicine but also in non-European medicine. In particular, folk medicine in premodern Korea manifests a belief that women receive needed energy or elements through their sexual/reproductive organs, due to those organs' openness. As in premodern Western medicine, the woman's body was understood as colder; consequently, women might need heat for managing general health and improving sexual/reproductive health. This understanding of the woman's body as colder and open seems to be shared between Korean traditional medicine and Hildegardian and other premodern European medicine.

Comparing Hildegard of Bingen's written voice with the cultural practices of Korean women demonstrates different methodological pathways for recovering women's contributions across diverse historical contexts. While Hildegard composed substantial written works on the basis of her own intellectual authority, although she received help from her male scribes, Korean women's cultural expression and writing did not receive the same authority and benefited from fewer opportunities to be considered scholarly. Korean women's own writings on medicine, in particular, have rarely survived. This contrast in documentary evidence necessitates different scholarly approaches: direct textual analysis in Hildegard's case versus interpretive reconstruction in the Korean context. Nevertheless, both investigations explore how women navigated patriarchal constraints while establishing their intellectual and cultural presence.

Particularly significant is how the concept of female bodily porosity, which is central to Hildegard's theological and medical understanding of women's reproductive and salvational roles, finds resonance across cultural boundaries. This porosity, which enabled women to receive, transform, and transmit both physical and spiritual elements in Hildegard's framework, offers a valuable interpretive tool for understanding Korean women's cultural mediations despite the patriarchal limitations they faced. Such transcultural perspectives help us to understand women's historical influence beyond conventional geographical and temporal boundaries, revealing how female embodiment itself has served as a site of creative expression and spiritual transformation as healing.

Along these lines, I will conclude my examination of women's understanding and practice of their porous bodies by shifting focus to analyze a specific medicinal herb: mugwort, or *Artemisia vulgaris* in its scientific nomenclature, along with the literature and practices surrounding its use. The Korean medicinal use of mugwort provides a useful case study of how concepts of female bodily porosity transcend cultural and temporal boundaries. This cross-cultural example reveals important parallels to medieval European understandings while demonstrating how women actively utilized their bodies' perceived permeability as a therapeutic pathway, especially when they could not expect help from male physicians. Just as Hildegard reframed female porosity from vulnerability to salvational potential, Korean women's medicinal practices show how perceived bodily openness became an opportunity for self-directed healing rather than merely a marker of inferiority.

Mugwort is one of the most popular medicinal herbs in many regions, including Europe, North America, Asia, and elsewhere, because it can easily survive in uncultivated areas. Mugwort is pervasively accessible and extensively employed in traditional practices and contemporary applications across Asia and Europe.[1] It was also used by medieval women, and Hildegard and the authors of the *Trotula* mentioned and recommended it. Playing a central role in herbology across different cultures, this herb has been believed to help human beings, and particularly women with women's health issues, throughout history.[2]

It should be also noted that mugwort is often confused with other similar herbs. Its scientific name, *Artemisia vulgaris*, is frequently misapplied, and historical records from both Eastern and Western traditions demonstrate that this designation was attached to various herbs, typically belonging to the *Artemisia* genus, which comprises more than five hundred species.[3] In Korea as well, 쑥 (*Ssuk*), the Korean name for mugwort, has been

---

1 Abiri et al., "Towards a Better Understanding of *Artemisia vulgaris*," 403.

2 Tobyn et al., *Western Herbal Tradition*, 123; Ekiert et al., "Significance of *Artemisia vulgaris* L. (Common Mugwort)," 4415.

3 For example, the name "mugwort" has been applied to wormwort (*Artemisia arborescens*), absinthe (*Artemisia absinthium*), sagebrush, field sagewort or tall wormwood (*Artemisia campetris*), sea wormwood (*Artemisia maritima*), and so on. What can be more challenging for modern researchers and readers is that the *Artemisia* genus is also confused with the *Tanacetum* genus, including tansy, and

applied to different kinds of *Artemisia*. Therefore, I do not attempt to strictly distinguish mugwort from similar herbs when they are understood as the same and used for the same purpose.

In the history of medicine in the West, mugwort was named the "mother of herbs" and known for helping mothers just as their friends would help them.[4] It was used externally to treat wounds, gout, and leg fatigue and internally to treat fever.[5] Importantly, it was believed that it could expel unwanted entities from a woman's body, such as menstrual blood, a dead foetus, or the placenta.

At the same time, mugwort is widely used in Asia, especially Korea. Mugwort has been historically and traditionally important in herbology, food, drink, and new drug development in Korea beginning in ancient times. This herb is used in many different ways in Korea and many countries in Asia. The most popular way is direct consumption. Mugwort can be taken alone or together with other food or drink. Known as a savoury, it is used as an ingredient in food. It can also be consumed as a beverage, either steeped as an herbal tea or ground into powder and mixed with other ingredients. Modern medicine has also recognized the value of this herb *and* used it to make cosmetics, health supplements, and air fresheners, as well as other medicinal uses. Recent studies have also investigated mugwort's potential as an antiparasitic and antimalarial agent.[6]

And one of the popular ways of using mugwort in Korea is fumigation treatment, in which the herb is dried and ground to be used in moxibustion. Moxibustion is the use of heat and smoke to treat patients and is popular in Eastern traditional medicine, including in China, Korea, Japan, Tibet, and Mongolia. While many different materials can be used for moxibustion, mugwort has been primarily used, beginning with ancient Chinese medicine.[7] The foundational belief is that moxibustion can circulate *qi* (or *chi*) 氣,[8] "ris-

---

the *Asteraceae* genus, which is believed to have similar characteristics of heat and could be substituted for mugwort. Even now, folk medicine does not particularly distinguish mugwort from similar herbs. Tobyn et al., *Western Herbal Tradition*, 125–26.

4 Black, *Medicine and Healing*, 221–22.

5 Ekiert et al., "Significance of *Artemisia vulgaris* L. (Common Mugwort)."

6 Kodippili et al., "Investigation of the Antimalarial Activity of *Artemisia vulgaris*," 276–81.

7 Yoeli-Tlalim, *Reorienting Histories of Medicine*, 88.

8 In Confucianism, *qi* is understood as vital energy and the embodiment of *li*, encompassing the more material components of the universe. Yin and yang were

ing vapor," so that it can deliver heat.[9] Moxibustion or moxa-cauterization can be traced in the manuscript tradition as far back as 168 BCE[10] and has played a prominent role in the field of Chinese medicine and Eastern Asian medicine influenced by it. However, it was not until the 1950s that this medical practice's efficacy was examined in the "scientific" method of the West.[11] According to traditional medicine, there are several ways to introduce smoke into the human body. While moxibustion can be applied directly to the skin, practitioners typically recommend performing this treatment near affected body parts. Additionally, the body possesses certain openings or import points considered gateways for needed energy. The navel represents a popular location for moxibustion, while the cervical opening serves as an ideal site for this treatment in women, highlighting the porosity of the female body and specifically women's reproductive organs.

Therefore, a particular method of fumigation treatment is recommended to women that is not practised on men in Korea. The basic logic is similar to other moxibustions in that it uses fumes, in particular mugwort smoke. The difference is that the smoke enters the woman's body directly, through the vagina. Dried mugwort is placed in a pot or any container with an opening on the top. The container with mugwort is then placed under a chair or a similar piece of furniture, on which a woman sits without clothing on the lower part of her body, covering her body as a whole with a long garment so that the smoke cannot escape. When the mugwort is burned, it gives off fumes or smoke. Modern methods of mugwort fumigation also use steam instead of smoke. This treatment can be easily found in Korean saunas and Korean medicine clinics.

In contemporary folk medicine in Korea, home care kits are available, too. It is commonly acknowledged that no physicians or specialists are required, and even women themselves can perform the procedure. Mugwort fumigation is expected to supply needed elements, that is, heat, to women. At the same time, mugwort smoke is also believed to kill bacteria or other harmful microorganisms.

---

produced out of *qi*, in complementary relations. The interaction, or even intercourse, between yin and yang, or the female and male powers, engenders the elements of the universe.

9 Unschuld, *Medicine in China*, 97.

10 Unschuld, *Medicine in China*, 93–94.

11 Liangyue, "Chinese Acupuncture and Moxibustion," 74–75.

In addition, Korean women can use mugwort in their sanitary pads.[12] Produced by several Korean companies, sanitary pads containing mugwort are a clear example of how the woman's body is understood as cold, on the side of yin, according to folk and traditional medicine supported by Taoism. By containing mugwort or its extract, the pad is supposed to supply heat to the woman's cold body. Simultaneously, pads containing mugwort are also believed to cover the odour from menstrual blood, helping women to conceal their periods. Whether or not mugwort actually works to bring fertility to women, modern Korean women who use it are making efforts to manage their own reproductive health, not necessarily depending on doctors and other medical personnel, who are likely male. Mugwort is also currently used for both men's and women's skincare, generally advertising its good effects on the skin of women, but for reproductive/sexual efficacy, mugwort is recommended only to women, not men.

Interestingly, mugwort fumigation was also recommended by ancient Western physicians, just like mugwort moxibustion in Asian medicine. For example, Paulus Aegineta knew and recommended fumigatory treatment with mugwort, which seems very similar to the Korean treatment that is still popular among women.

> In dealing with cases of sterility, our author says that when the mouth of the uterus is shut up, it must be opened by injections of aromatics and by using fomentation. Fumigations of the womb may be applied either by sitting on a proper chair, and receiving the vapours which arise, or by injections of hot water in which safe, mugwort, rue, cumin, pennyroyal, sweet flag, and the aromatic seeds, have been boiled.[13]

Here, mugwort is used in the form of smoke or in hot water. Both methods were believed to deliver mugwort to the uterus, where the woman suffers from infertility. The smoke or water was to be inserted into the woman's body, where it was believed to open the closed uterus, possibly with the heat that mugwort and hot water were considered to have. Different herbs used along with mugwort were also considered hot by nature. Beyond its gynae-

---

12 Youngjoo Lee 이영주. "Ilhoeyong saengridaeui doipgwa wolgyeonghaneun mom-e daehan insik-ui byeonhwa: 1960–1980 nyeondae Hanguk-ui gyeongu" 일회용 생리대의 도입과 월경하는 몸에 대한 인식의 변화 : 1960–1980 년대 한국의 경우 [The Introduction of Disposable Menstrual Products and the Change of Perception about the Menstrual Body], 1.

13 McKay, *History of Ancient Gynaecology*, 228.

cological uses, mugwort was also worn by men and animals to drive away evil spirits.[14]

The *Trotula* also recommends to female patients a mugwort fumigatory treatment that is surprisingly similar to Korean women's way of using this herb. Again, this treatment uses mugwort smoke in the belief that it will enter the woman's vagina and reach the uterus. Fumigatory treatment can be performed through the nose and umbilicus for both women and men, but the application to the reproductive organs is only for women.[15] As described in the chapter on retention of the menses in the *Trotula*, medieval mugwort fumigatory treatment sends mugwort smoke to the lower part of the female patient so that her body can be exposed to it and can absorb the smoke.[16] Also, in the section "On Paucity of the Menses" in the same book, the author introduces another fumigation treatment, using ginger, laurel leaves, and savin. The method is the same. The practitioner is to prepare the herbs as powders and burn them in a pot while a woman "sits upon a perforated seat" in order to receive "the smoke through the lower members" to bring on full menstruation. Other herbs in addition to mugwort can be used with slightly different treatments: "Likewise, chickweed cooked in an earthenware pot and placed over [the belly] provokes the menses."[17]

In the medieval West, fumigation treatment was also used when the woman's womb was descended, the prolapse of the womb, which traces back to Roman medicine.[18] In the premodern period, many physicians believed that the womb could move within the woman's body, causing various health issues. The *Trotula* diagnoses that this descent of the womb could occur due to weak bodily members and abundant cold humours and could possibly be cured by a fumigatory treatment that was preceded and followed by many other cures.

---

14 Armstrong, "Mugwort Lore," 22.

15 Fumigation treatment was also used in the Roman treatment for phrenitis, using wool. Black, *Medicine and Healing*, 98.

16 Fumigatory treatment was also used to check a woman's fertility. In premodern medicine, it was believed that fumigation was useful in that the smoke could reach the troubled woman's womb directly. If the fumes did not pass into the woman's body, especially the vagina and the womb, it means that her body was blocked and possibly unable to have a child. Evans, "Female Barrenness, Bodily Access and Aromatic Treatments," 424–43.

17 Green, trans., *The Trotula*, 79.

18 Pliny the Elder recommends fumigation with wool in the case of the womb's prolapse. Black, *Medicine and Healing*, 99.

> Then let there be made for them a steambath, which works very well. For Dioscorides prescribes that there be made for them a steambath of box wood placed in a pot upon live coals, and let the woman, covered on top, sit on it, and let her receive the smoke inside [her vagina].[19]

Although the efficacy is different, the fumigation treatment is conducted in the same way. Instead of mugwort, burning coals are used. The interesting thing is that this treatment is believed to help patients only when their pain is caused by coldness of the body. If cramps are caused by excessive heat, the treatments are different, because the pain comes from the womb being immoderately dry and hot.[20] From the fact that coals can be used instead of mugwort in this treatment, we can reasonably infer that the fumes were believed to convey heat and that the fumigatory treatment can transmit the fumes and their heat.

Where mugwort is concerned, it should be noted that this herb was regarded as having heating properties in medieval Western medicine, just as in the Korean pharmaceutical tradition. Medieval European writers classified mugwort as an herb with a hot nature. Hildegard was no exception, similarly categorizing mugwort as "very hot" in her *Physica*, recommending it for warming a "cold stomach" just as Korean medicine prescribes it to balance women's cold nature. This parallel classification across distant medical traditions suggests a remarkably consistent conceptualization of both herbal properties and female bodily needs.

> Mugwort (*biboz*) is very hot, and its juice is of very great value. If it is cooked and eaten as a puree, it heals ailing intestines and warms a cold stomach. But, if someone eats or drinks something which has given *them* pain, then *they* should cook and eat warmed mugwort with meat or lard, or as a puree, or with any other condiment. It will attract the rotten matter which was in the previously ingested food or drink, and chase it away. If bad humors gather in some part of the body, flowing out from broken skin where there is no poisoned wound, the person should take mugwort and express the juice. To the juice *they* should add a smaller amount of honey. *They* should spread this on the afflicted area, then cover it with egg white, and tie it with a cloth. *They* should do this until *they are* better.[21]

19 Green, trans., *The Trotula*, 87–89.

20 Green, trans., *The Trotula*, 157.

21 Modified from Hildegard of Bingen, *Physica*, trans. Throop, 56. In the English quotation block, I use italics to indicate modifications I have made to the pronouns used in the English translation cited. However, the following Latin passage preserves the italics as they appear in the original manuscript: "*Biboz* [Artemisia *ed.*] valde calida est, et succus ejus valde utilis; et si coquitur et in *muse* comeditur, infirma

Due to its hot nature, mugwort was understood to cure symptoms caused by excessive coldness, especially gynaecological issues. This belief is also seen in premodern Western academic medicine, but in this context, women developed their own ways of taking care of their bodies, including midwifery, which was often dismissed in the written male medical tradition.

The persistence of mugwort in contemporary Korean women's health practices demonstrates how ancient ideas about female bodies endure and are adapted across centuries, much as Hildegard's positive reframing of female porosity continued to influence medieval European understandings of women's reproductive health. When examined across cultural boundaries, these parallel traditions demonstrate both convergences and divergences that invite fresh analytical approaches. The temporal and conceptual irregularities that emerge within a comparative framework generate productive tensions that allow scholars to formulate more nuanced research questions and reach innovative conclusions about women's bodily knowledge.[22] In both cases, women transformed potentially limiting conceptions of their physiology into pragmatic healing practices.

This project opened with a discussion of medieval medical traditions in Europe that described women's bodies as having qualities of coldness and that viewed women's bodies as more porous, permeable, and breakable than men's bodies. Female physiological cycles (menstruation) and shapes (the womb's concave appearance) seemed to support these ideas. The book then moved from the reception of female biology to discuss religious accounts that represent women's physical porosity allegorically. Medieval theology and church teachings both praised women (for their humility, as in the Virgin's pregnancy) and condemned them (as easily breakable and transgres-

---

viscera sanat, ac stomachum frigidum calefacit. Sed et si quis comederit aut biberit, unde dolet, tunc aut ex carnibus, aut cum sagimine, aut in *muse*, aut in aliquo alio condimento et temperamento *biboz* coquat et comedat, et putredinem hanc quam in prioribus cibis aut potibus ille sibi attraxit aufert et fugat. Sed et si troffo, et mali humores, rupta cute absque venenato ulcere in aliquo loco corporis humani coadunati effluunt, homo ille artemisiam accipiat, et exprimat, et eidem succo mel addat, ita ut succus artemisiae mel excedat, et sic locum doloris perungat. Mox etiam clarum de albugine ovi factum superilliniat, et panno desuper liget. Et hoc tam diu faciat dum sanetur." Hildegard of Bingen, *Physica*, bk. 1, chap. 107, in Hildegard of Bingen, *S. Hildegardis Abbatissae Opera omnia*, §§1171–72.

22 On new approaches and new conclusions in comparative research on understanding women's culture, see McAvoy and Niebrzydowski, "Introduction: Medieval Women's Literary Cultures," 13.

sive, as in Eve's actions in Paradise), which lent support and authority to the physiological ideas, theories, and knowledge about women of the time.

In the theological understanding of physiology, which was related to the appearance and function of women's reproductive bodies, women were often referred to as vessels, in the religious sense that women could relatively easily be filled with holy or evil spirits. This notion of women as porous vessels is also related to Eve, who was the first woman and the unsealer of sin. The most visible symptoms of women's porous bodies, namely menstruation and childbirth, however, were often treated as pollutants and were even used to justify limits on women's activities.

In contrast, Hildegard of Bingen discovered possibilities of purgation and salvation in the woman's porous body. In her medical book, *Cause et cure*, she interprets women's permeable bodies, especially the womb, as capable of flexibility and correct balance. Interestingly, in her theological work *Scivias*, Hildegard uses this strong understanding of women's physical permeability to present Ecclesia's capacity for purging souls and giving humanity new life. Her positive depictions in her spiritual writings are deeply indebted to her gynaecological knowledge and were bolstered by her understanding of the womb and women's reproductive processes as purgative and redemptive, rather than polluting and inferior.

This book is not an all-encompassing study intended to discover the hidden history of the woman's body and understandings of it. Rather, it is a starting point for suggesting new approaches to broaden an important step in understanding women's health. When the definition and application of medicine are widened to incorporate women's own practices to take care of their bodies, increase their fertility, and eliminate health issues, women become better able to manage their own bodies.

The shared belief that the woman's body is porous and permeable, common in many cultures, was seen as an opportunity by some women. For Hildegard, menstrual flow, pregnancy, and childbirth show the woman's possibility to purge, heal, and save humankind, based on the beauty of weakness. Just as many medieval European gynaecological writings prescribe treatments to women using their body's porosity, traditional Korean women also find ways to heal their reproductive issues by absorbing mugwort fumes through their vaginas, believed to be open.

While it is true that many "womanly" diseases were understood as limited to sexual and reproductive issues, it is still valid that many women suffered from them. And many issues were explained through their lack of heat, something already prevalent in the understanding of sex/gender differences in premodern European and premodern Korean cultures. Menstruation, which is directly related to women's fertility, depends on the balance of heat and coldness. In general, menstruation retention is explained by cold wind in Asia and excessive coldness in Europe.

At the same time, women could find cures for themselves or from other women. While they could ask for professional help from male physicians, they could also use mugwort, which could be easily found in their neighbourhood or fields, and apply its fumes to their reproductive organs. If a woman's body was sick or infertile due to a lack of heat, they could supply the needed heat. The fumes will enter their bodies through the openings of the reproductive organs that were already assumed to exist. In this way, porosity becomes an opportunity for healing.

It should be noted that Hildegard of Bingen emphasized that she herself was porous. Hildegard of Bingen was also a woman, and she commented on her own weak nature and porous body. She was called a "fragile vessel" by her biographers. She called herself "unlearned." Her demure presentation of her own gender also appears in her letters.

As always, however, Hildegard of Bingen turned her weak points into strong points. Hildegard recorded the *Scivias* in order to remind male theologians and priests that they were not obeying God's will. Hildegard referred to her time as an "effeminate age" many times in her letters,[23] signalling her sense that the men of her time had lost their way: "Wisdom cries out, saying: The present time is a squalid, womanish time."[24] And that is why she considered women in the vanguard of God's work: "This time is a womanish time, because the dispensation of God's justice is weak. But the strength of God's justice is exerting itself, a female warrior battling against injustice, so that it might fall defeated."[25] This idea was also discussed by Elizabeth of Schönau, Hildegard's spiritual friend and protégée, who presented it more directly in her *Liber visionum*, pointing to the female prophets of the Old Testament for support.

---

23 Baird and Ehrman, "Introduction," 12.

24 "Hildegard to Hillinus, Archbishop of Trier," in Hildegard of Bingen, *Letters*, trans. Baird and Ehrman, no. 26r, 1:88. Hildegard did not use the "effeminate age" as a positive characterization but as a negative one, sarcastically, as Barbara Newman elaborates. However, at the same time, Hildegard used this term to justify the existence of women leaders because authoritative men have already become "effeminate." Newman, *Sister of Wisdom*, 239.

25 "Hildegard to the Prelates at Mainz," in Hildegard of Bingen, *Letters*, trans. Baird and Ehrman, no. 23, 1:79.

> People are scandalized that in these days the Lord deigns to magnify his great mercy in the frail sex. But why doesn't it cross their minds that a similar thing happened in the days of our fathers when, while men were given to indolence, holy women were filled with the Spirit of God so that they could prophesy, energetically govern the people of God, and even win glorious victories over Israel's enemies? I speak of women like Hilda, Deborah, Judith, Jael, and the like.[26]

Teaching and preaching God's words were first and foremost men's duties. However, since they were neglecting their duties, God wanted this weak woman, Hildegard, to be his prophet, to spread his message, and to correct men's misbehaviour. Hildegard placed herself in a genealogy of prophets descending from the Old Testament, who had also challenged authority by proclaiming that their religious leaders were not listening to God. Moreover, this reversal of conventional power dynamics was also applicable to Jesus, who chose to become a weak and lowly human being to save humanity. "But God hath chosen the foolish things of the world to confound the wise; and God hath chosen the weak things of the world to confound the things which are mighty; And base things of the world, and things which are despised, hath God chosen, yea, and things which are not, to bring to nought things that are: That no flesh should glory in his presence" (1 Corinthians 1:27–29).

While medieval theology taught that Mary was the holy window of salvation who received the Holy Spirit, and Ecclesia represented the female body's ability to cleanse sin from people's souls, Hildegard was God's messenger, who received his words in visions, put them into writing, interpreted the female body in a positive light, and represented women's reproductive role as salvational, purgative, and God-like.

26 Translation from Newman, *Sister of Wisdom*, 39. "Hoc illos scandalizat, quod in his diebus plurimum in sexu fragili misericordiam suam dominus magnificare dignatur. Sed cur in mentem non venit, quoniam simile factum est in diebus patrum nostrorum, quando viris socordie deditis, spiritu dei replete sunt mulieres sancte, ut prophetarent, populum dei strennue gubernarent, sive etiam de hostibus Israel gloriose triumpharent, quemadmodum Olda, Debora, Judith, Jahel, et huiusmodi?" Elizabeth of Schönau, *Liber visionum secundus I*, ed. Roth, bk. 2, chap. 1, p. 40.

BIBLIOGRAPHY

Primary Sources

Aristotle. *De generatione animalium*. Translated by Arthur Platt. Clarendon, 1910.

Elizabeth of Schönau. "Liber visionum secundus I." In *Die Visionen der hl. Elisabeth und die Schriften der Äbte Ekbert und Emecho von Schönau*. Edited by F. W. E. Roth, 40–55. Brünn, 1884.

Galen. *On the Usefulness of the Parts of the Body*. Translated by Margaret Tallmadge. Cornell University Press, 1968.

Gratian. *The Treatise on Laws (Decretum DD. 1–20)*. Translated by Augustine Thompson. With the Ordinary Gloss translated by James Gordley and an Introduction by Katherine Christensen. Studies in Medieval and Early Modern Canon Law 2. Catholic University of America Press, 1993.

Gregory the Great. *Registrum epistolarum*. Translated by James Barmby. In *Nicene and Post-Nicene Fathers*, 2nd ser., vol. 13. Edited by Henry Wace and Philip Schaff. Christian Literature, 1898. Revised and edited for New Advent by Kevin Knight. New Advent. https://www.newadvent.org/fathers/360211064.htm.

Green, Monica H., trans. *The Trotula: A Medieval Compendium of Women's Medicine*. University of Pennsylvania Press, 2001.

Hildegard of Bingen. *Analecta sacra spicilegio Solesmes*, vol. 8, *Hildegardis Opera*. Edited by Jean Baptiste Pitra. Jouby et Roger, 1882.

——. *Beate Hildegardis Cause et cure*. Edited by Laurence Moulinier and Rainer Berndt. Akademie, 2003.

——. *Book of Divine Works*. Translated by Nathaniel M Campbell. The Catholic University of America Press, 2016.

——. *Causes and Cures: The Complete English Translation of "Hildegardis Causae et curae: Libri VI."* Translated by Priscilla Throop. MedievalMS, 2008.

——. *Hildegard of Bingen's Book of Divine Works: With Letters and Songs*. Edited by Matthew Fox. Inner Traditions/Bear, 1987.

——. *Hildegardis Causae et curae*. Edited by Paul Kaiser. Teubner, 1903.

——. *Homilies on the Gospels*. Translated by Beverly Mayne Kienzle. Liturgical Press, 2011.

——. *The Letters of Hildegard of Bingen*. 3 vols. Translated by Joseph L. Baird and Radd K. Ehrman. Oxford University Press, 1998–2004.

——. *Liber divinorum operum*. Edited by Albert Derolez and Peter Dronke. Corpus Christianorum Continuatio Mediaevalis 92. Brepols, 1996.

——. *Physica: The Complete English Translation of Her Classic Work on Health and Healing*. Translated by Priscilla Throop. Healing Arts, 1998.

——. *S. Hildegardis Abbatissae Opera omnia, ad optimorum librorum fidem edita*. Edited by Jacques-Paul Migne. Patrologiae cursus completus: Series latina 197. Paris, 1855. Reprint, Brepols, 1976.

——. *Scivias*. Edited by Adelgundis Führkötter and Angela Carelvaris. Corpus Christianorum Continuatio Mediaevalis 43. Brepols, 1978.

——. *Scivias*. Translated by Columba Hart and Jane Bishop. Classics of Western Spirituality. Paulist Press, 1990.

Honorius. *The Seal of Blessed Mary*. Translated by Amelia Carr. Peregrina, 1991.

Isidore of Seville. *Isidori Hispalensis Episcopi Etymologiarum sive originum libri XX*. Vol. 1, *Libros I–X continens*. Edited by W. M. Lindsay. Oxford University Press, 1911.

Paucapalea. *Die Summa des Paucapalea über das Decretum Gratiani*. Edited by Johann Friedrich von Schulte. Giessen, 1890.

Peter Lombard. *The Sentences: Book 2 on Creation*. Translated by Giulio Silano. Mediaeval Sources in Translation. Pontifical Institute of Mediaeval Studies, 2007.

Pseudo-Albertus Magnus. *De secretis mulierum libellus*. Lyon: Ioannes Quadratus, 1580. Munich, Bayerische Staatsbibliothek, Anat. 17. Münchener Digitalisierungs-Zentrum Digitale Bibliothek, https://www.digitale-sammlungen.de/en/view/bsb10172791.

——. *El "De secretis mulierum" atribuido a Alberto Magno: Estudio, edición crítica y traducción*. Translated by José Pablo Barragán Nieto. Textes et études du Moyen Âge 63. Fédération internationale des Instituts d'études médiévales, 2012.

——. *Women's Secrets: A Translation of Pseudo-Albertus Magnus' "De secretis mulierum" with Commentaries*. Translated by Helen Rodnite Lemay. State University of New York Press, 1992.

Rufinus. *Summa decretorum*. Edited by Heinrich Singer. Schöningh, 1902. Reprint, Scientia, 1963.

Thomas Aquinas. *Summa theologiae*. Translated by the Fathers of the English Dominican Province. 2nd rev. ed. 1920. Online edition by Kevin Knight. New Advent, 2017. https://www.newadvent.org/summa.

Vita Sanctae Hildegardis. Edited by Monica Klaes. Corpus Christianorum Continuatio Mediaevalis 126. Brepols, 1993.

Secondary Studies

Abiri, Rambod, Abraão Lincoln Macedo Silva, Ludmilla Santos Silva de Mesquita, et al. "Towards a Better Understanding of *Artemisia vulgaris*: Botany, Phytochemistry, Pharmacological and Biotechnological Potential." *Food Research International* 109 (July 2018): 403–15.

Armstrong, Edward A. "Mugwort Lore." *Folklore* 55, no. 1 (1944): 22–27.

Baird, Joseph L., and Radd K. Ehrman. "Introduction." In Hildegard of Bingen, *The Letters of Hildegard of Bingen*, translated by Joseph L. Baird and Radd K. Ehrman, 1:3–26. Oxford University Press, 1998.

Barnes, W. R., Rebecca Hayward, Kathleen Loncar, and Michael Wright. *Writing the Wilton Women: Goscelin's Legend of Edith and Liber confortatorius*. Brepols, 2004.

Black, Winston. *Medicine and Healing in the Premodern West: A History in Documents*. Broadview, 2019.

Blumenfeld-Kosinski, Renate. "Visions and Schism Politics in the Twelfth Century: Hildegard of Bingen, John of Salisbury, and Elisabeth of Schönau." In *Saints, Scholars, and Politicians: Gender as a Tool in Medieval Studies*, edited by Mathilde van Dijk and Renée Nip, 173–87. Brepols, 2005.

Bradley, Mark. *Colour and Meaning in Ancient Rome*. Cambridge Classical Studies. Cambridge University Press, 2009.

Bullough, Vern L. "Marriage in the Middle Ages: Medieval Medical and Scientific Views of Women." *Viator* 4 (1973): 485–501.

Bynum, Caroline Walker. "'...And Woman His Humanity': Female Imagery in the Religious Writing of the Later Middle Ages." In *Gender and Religion: On the Complexity of Symbols*, edited by Caroline Walker Bynum, Stevan Harrel, and Paula Richman, 257–88. Beacon, 1986.

——. *Holy Feast and Holy Fast: The Religious Significance of Food to Medieval Women*. New Historicism. University of California Press, 1987.

——. *Wonderful Blood: Theology and Practice in Late Medieval Northern Germany and Beyond*. University of Pennsylvania Press, 2007.

Caciola, Nancy. *Discerning Spirits: Divine and Demonic Possession in the Middle Ages*. Cornell University Press, 2003.

Cadden, Joan. "It Takes All Kinds: Sexuality and Gender Differences in Hildegard of Bingen's 'Book of Compound Medicine.'" *Traditio* 40 (1984): 149–74.

——. *Meanings of Sex Difference in the Middle Ages: Medicine, Science, and Culture*. Cambridge University Press, 1993.

Campbell, Nathaniel M. "The Prophetess and the Pope: St. Hildegard of Bingen, Pope Benedict XVI, and Prophetic Visions of Church Reform." In *Prophetic Futures*, edited by Joseph Bowling and Katherine Walker, 21–34. Springer, 2023.

Charmaille, Françoise. "Intersex between Sex and Gender in *Cause et cure*." *Exemplaria* 33 (2021): 327–43.

Constas, Nicholas. *Proclus of Constantinople and the Cult of the Virgin in Late Antiquity: Homilies 1–5, Texts and Translations*. Brill, 2003.

Corrigan, Vincent J. "Hildegard of Bingen." In *Icons of the Middle Ages: Rulers, Writers, Rebels, and Saints*, edited by Lister M. Matheson, 2:355–94. Bloomsbury, 2011.

Crowther, Katherine M. *Adam and Eve in the Protestant Reformation*. Cambridge University Press, 2010.

DeVun, Leah. "Erecting Sex: Hermaphrodites and the Medieval Science of Surgery." *Osiris* 30, no. 1 (2015): 17–37.

Duden, Barbara. *The Woman Beneath the Skin: A Doctor's Patients in Eighteenth-Century Germany*. Harvard University Press, 1991.

Ekiert, Halina, Joanna Pajor, Paweł Klin, Agnieszka Rzepiela, Halina Ślesak, and Agnieszka Szopa. "Significance of *Artemisia vulgaris* L. (Common Mugwort) in the History of Medicine and Its Possible Contemporary Applications Substantiated by Phytochemical and Pharmacological Studies." *Molecules* 25, no. 19 (2020): 4415.

Elliot, Dyan. "Gender and the Christian Traditions." In *The Oxford Handbook of Women and Gender in Medieval Europe*, edited by Judith M. Bennett and Ruth Mazo Karras, 21–35. Oxford University Press, 2013.

Embach, Michael. "The Life of Hildegard of Bingen (1098–1179)." In *The Cambridge Companion to Hildegard of Bingen*, edited by Jennifer Bain, 11–36. Cambridge University Press, 2021.

Evans, Jennifer. "Female Barrenness, Bodily Access and Aromatic Treatments in Seventeenth-Century England." *Historical Research* 87 (2014): 424–43.

Fassler, Margot E. *Cosmos, Liturgy, and the Arts in the Twelfth Century: Hildegard's Illuminated "Scivias."* University of Pennsylvania Press, 2023.

Feiss, Hugh. "Introduction." In *Two Hagiographies: Vita Sancti Rupperti Confessoris and Vita Sancti Dysibodi Episcopi*. Edited by Christopher P. Evans, translated by Hugh Feiss, 1–32. Dallas Medieval Texts and Translations 11. Peeters, 2010.

Green, Monica H. "From 'Diseases of Women' to 'Secrets of Women': The Transformation of Gynecological Literature in the Later Middle Ages." *Journal of Medieval and Early Modern Studies* 30 (2000): 5–39.

——. "In Search of an 'Authentic' Women's Medicine: The Strange Fates of Trota of Salerno and Hildegard of Bingen." *Dynamis: Acta hispanica ad medicinae scientiarumque historiam illustrandam* 19 (1999): 25–54.

——. *Making Women's Medicine Masculine: The Rise of Male Authority in Pre-Modern Gynaecology*. Oxford University Press, 2008.

Hayton, Magda. "Hildegardian Prophecy and French Prophecy Collections, 1378–1455: A Study and Critical Edition of the 'Schism Extracts.'" *Traditio* 72 (2017): 453–91.

Irigaray, Luce. *Speculum of the Other Woman*. Translated by Gillian C. Gill. Cornell University Press, 1985.

Jacquart, Danielle, and Claude Alexandre Thomasset. *Sexuality and Medicine in the Middle Ages*. Translated by Matthew Adamson. Princeton University Press, 1988.

Kalas, Laura. "Hildegard's *Causae et curae*." In *The Palgrave Encyclopedia of Medieval Women's Writing in the Global Middle Ages*, edited by Michaelle M. Sauer, Diane Watt, and Liz Herbert McAvoy, 1–3. Palgrave Macmillan, 2023.

Karras, Ruth Mazo. *Sexuality in Medieval Europe: Doing unto Others*. Routledge, 2012.

Kerby-Fulton, Kathryn. "Prophet and Reformer: 'Smoke in the Vineyard.'" In *Voice of the Living Light: Hildegard of Bingen and Her World*, edited by Barbara Newman, 70–90. University of California Press, 1998.

Kienzle, Beverly Mayne. "Introduction." In Hildegard of Bingen, *Homilies on the Gospels*, translated by Beverly Mayne Kienzle, 1–28. Cistercian Studies Series 241. Cistercian Publications, 2011.

Kodippili, Kasun, Wanigasekera Daya Ratnasooriya, Sirimal Premakumara, and Preethi V. Udagama. "An Investigation of the Antimalarial Activity of *Artemisia vulgaris* Leaf Extract in a Rodent Malaria Model." *International Journal of Green Pharmacy* 5, no. 4 (2011): 276–81.

Koren, Sharon Faye. "The Menstruant as 'Other' in Medieval Judaism and Christianity." *Nashim: A Journal of Jewish Women's Studies and Gender Issues* 17 (2009): 33–59.

Kruger, Steven F. "Becoming Christian, Becoming Male?" In *Becoming Male in the Middle Ages*, edited by Jeffrey Jerome Cohen and Bonnie Wheeler, 21–41. Garland, 1997. Reprint Routledge, 2015.

Langum, Virginia. *Medicine and the Seven Deadly Sins in Late Medieval Literature and Culture*. The New Middle Ages. Palgrave Macmillan, 2016.

Laqueur, Thomas. *Making Sex: Body and Gender from the Greeks to Freud*. Harvard University Press, 1992.

Lee, Minji. "The Womb in Labour: Representing the Woman's Body as an Active Vessel in Hildegard of Bingen's *Cause et cure*." *Social History of Medicine* 35, no. 4 (2022): 1183–99.

Lee Youngjoo 이영주. "Ilhoeyong saengridaeui doipgwa wolgyeonghaneun mom-e daehan insik-ui byeonhwa: 1960–1980 nyeondae Hanguk-ui gyeongu" 일회용 생리대의 도입과 월경하는 몸에 대한 인식의 변화 : 1960–1980 년대 한국의 경우 [The Introduction of Disposable Menstrual Products and the Change of Perception about the Menstrual Body]." MA Thesis, Seoul National University, 2018.

Lemay, Helen Rodnite. "Introduction." In Pseudo-Albertus Magnus, *Women's Secrets: A Translation of Pseudo-Albertus Magnus's "De secretis mulierum" with Commentaries*, translated by Helen Rodnite Lemay, 1–58. State University of New York Press, 1992.

Liangyue, Deng. "Chinese Acupuncture and Moxibustion." In *Traditional Medicine in Asia*, edited by Ranjit Roy Chaudhury and Uton Muchtar Rafei. 75–91. World Health Organization Regional Office for South-East Asia, 2001.

Lochrie, Karma. *Heterosyncrasies: Female Sexuality When Normal Wasn't*. New ed. University of Minnesota Press, 2005.

Loewen, Peter V. "From the Root to the Branches: Greenness in the Preaching of Hildegard of Bingen and the Patriarchs." In *The Cambridge Companion to Hildegard of Bingen*, edited by Jennifer Bain, 125–69. Cambridge Companions to Literature. Cambridge University Press, 2021.

Matter, E. Ann. *The Voice of My Beloved: The Song of Songs in Western Medieval Christianity*. The Middle Ages Series. University of Pennsylvania Press, 2010.

McAvoy, Liz Herbert. *The Enclosed Garden and the Medieval Religious Imaginary*. Brewer, 2021.

McAvoy, Liz Herbert, and Sue Niebrzydowski. "Introduction: Medieval Women's Literary Cultures and Thinking Beyond the Local." In *Women's Literary Cultures in the Global Middle Ages: Speaking Internationally*, edited by Kathryn Loveridge, Liz Herbert McAvoy, Vicki Kay Price, and Sue Niebrzydowski, 1–20. Boydell & Brewer, 2023.

McKay, William John Steward. *The History of Ancient Gynaecology*. Baillière, Tindall, and Cox, 1901.

Mews, Constant J. "Hildegard and the Schools." In *Hildegard of Bingen: The Context of Her Thought and Art*, edited by Charles Burnett and Peter Dronke, 89–110. Warburg Institute Colloquia 4. Warburg Institute, 1998.

Miles, Laura Saetveit. *The Virgin Mary's Book at the Annunciation: Reading, Interpretation, and Devotion in Medieval England*. Brewer, 2020.

Miles, Margaret R. *Carnal Knowing: Female Nakedness and Religious Meaning in the Christian West*. Wipf & Stock, 2006.

Moulinier, Laurence, and Rainer Berndt. "Introduction." In Hildegard of Bingen, *Beate Hildegardis Cause et cure*, edited by Laurence Moulinier and Rainer Berndt, xi–cxiii. Akademie, 2003.

Murray, Jacqueline. "One Flesh, Two Sexes, Three Genders?" In *Gender and Christianity in Medieval Europe: New Perspectives*, edited by Lisa M. Bitel and Felice Lifshitz, 34–51. University of Pennsylvania Press, 2008.

Newman, Barbara. *God and the Goddesses: Vision, Poetry, and Belief in the Middle Ages*. University of Pennsylvania Press, 2003.

——. "Hildegard and Her Hagiographers: The Remaking of Female Sainthood." In *Gendered Voices: Medieval Saints and Their Interpreters*, edited by Catherine M. Mooney, 16–34. University of Pennsylvania Press, 1999.

——. "Introduction." In Hildegard of Bingen, *Scivias*, translated by Columba Hart and Jane Bishop, 9–53. Paulist Press, 1990.

——. *Sister of Wisdom: St. Hildegard's Theology of the Feminine*. University of California Press, 1998.

Power, Marla N. "Menstruation and Reproduction: An Oglala Case." *Signs* 6, no. 1 (1980): 54–65.

Raming, Ida. *A History of Women and Ordination*. Vol. 2, *The Priestly Office of Women: God's Gift to a Renewed Church*. Edited and translated by Bernard Cooke and Gary Macy. Scarecrow, 2002.

Rapp, Beverlee Sian. "A Woman Speaks: Language and Self-Representation in Hildegard's Letters." In *Hildegard of Bingen: A Book of Essays*, edited by Maud Burnett McInerney, 3–24. Garland Medieval Casebooks 20. Routledge, 1998.

Rubin, Miri. *Mother of God: A History of the Virgin Mary*. Yale University Press, 2009.

Salih, Sarah. *Versions of Virginity in Late Medieval England*. Brewer, 2001.

Smoller, Laura Ackerman. *History, Prophecy, and the Stars: The Christian Astrology of Pierre d'Ailly, 1350–1420*. Princeton University Press, 1994.

Sur, Carolyn Wörman. *The Feminine Images of God in the Visions of Saint Hildegard of Bingen's "Scivias."* Mellen, 1993.

Sweet, Victoria. *Rooted in the Earth, Rooted in the Sky: Hildegard of Bingen and Premodern Medicine*. Studies in Medieval History and Culture. Routledge, 2006.

Tobyn, Graeme, Alison Denham, and Midge Whitelegg. *The Western Herbal Tradition: 2000 Years of Medicinal Plant Knowledge*. Kingsley, 2016.

Unschuld, Paul Ulrich. *Medicine in China: A History of Pharmaceutics*. University of California Press, 1986.

Vaughan, Theresa A. *Women, Food, and Diet in the Middle Ages: Balancing the Humours*. Amsterdam University Press, 2020.

Yoeli-Tlalim, Ronit. *Reorienting Histories of Medicine: Encounters along the Silk Roads*. Bloomsbury Academic, 2021.

York, William H. *Health and Wellness in Antiquity Through the Middle Ages*. Greenwood, 2012.

INDEX